Consequences of Diagnostic Errors on Patient Safety

Richard P. Gusman

Abstract

The purpose for this qualitative research was to provide comparative data to determine if there was areas in need of improvement when it pertained to medical errors. Researchers have validated that initiating measures for continuous improvement would minimize error rates and benefit the clinicians and their patients. Patient safety was important and cause major concerns, therefore this research explored categories that influenced decision-making processes or conditions that causes deficit in reasoning, which could have an impact on cognitive abilities. Therefore, medical errors are a research worthy problem; since they cause phenomenon, conflict within managerial processes, and was a contributing factor for malpractice payouts, per a report from 2015 Institute of Medicine. As a result, researchers validated that initiating measures for continuous improvement would benefit the clinicians and their patients by minimizing errors or keeping them at a minimum. Utilizing the qualitative approach provided the best framework to narrow down cause and effects to validate the importance of support that relates to memory and relational network through retrieval-mediated learning. This research provides evidence that medical errors occurred during decision-making processes with (90%) cognitive errors, anchoring (75.7%), and (78.6%) premature closure. As a result, this qualitative research concentrated on constructs, such as, data collection from observation of prior research from scholarly, empirical, peered reviewed articles; *Medical Journals*, and education materials to provide pertinent information on diagnostic medical errors for the material within this investigation. The results from this study indicated, although, there was suggestions to improve patient-safety no significant decrease in medical harm occurred, therefore additional investigations will provide a valuable contribution to the body of knowledge and conditions for

continuous improvement.

Table of Contents

Chapter 1: Introduction

According to previous studies, patient safety was not on the medical profession's priority list when it pertained to preventing medical errors; although no exact number was proven. In addition, reluctance to report mistakes and/or inaccuracies in medical record errors continued to increase (Allen, & Pierce, 2016). This was causing great concerns for the medical profession, primarily, due to areas where moral concerns and ethics were questionable; therefore, one might ask how massive the errors were. According, to research from 2016 data verified diagnostic errors accounted for 17% of preventable errors for those patients hospitalized; approximately 9% of patients experience major undetected diagnostic errors while they were alive. In addition, per a Harvard Medical Practice study thousands of patients hospitalized died every year, because of diagnostic errors and physician-patient communication (Dass-Brailsford, deMendoza, Giller, Green, Power, Saunders, Schelbert, & Wisson, 2016; Patient Safety Network, 2016). This research provides information that focused on removing issues that was attributed to bias and associated with heuristics, in the category of diagnostic impression that derive from placing undue reliance on expert opinion or total reliance on test results. This process streamlined error rates by providing information that focus on patients, families, and the importance of integrity in the health-care profession (Fins, & Stark, 2014; Patient Safety Network, 2016). Furthermore, concerns about patient safety and medical doctors having sufficient training has been on the rise over the past decade and it has drawn attention to quantified and qualitative problems that pertain to medical errors, post-surgical complications, and health-care associated infections (Bass-Brailsford et al. 2016). Furthermore, there was evidence from previous studies that indicates complex interventions may be associated with qualitative and/or quantitative issues or occurrences (Higgins, Mayhew, Noyes, Pantoja, Petticrew, Rehfuess, Shemilt, & Sowden, 2013). Therefore, this study provides construct that consist of qualitative data composed in a cross-cultural context to synthesize evidence that causes complex interventions to become questionable and result in medical errors, along with validating areas that was in need of improvement. In addition, the study provides evidence that the quality of health care was continuously improving in comparison to data from the years of 2012 through 2017. The end results for this study provides data that consist of qualitative information, since quality was a major concern for both practitioner and patients. Utilizing the qualitative approach provided additional information that was pertinent for identifying causes for medical errors, so the data indicates the quality of care before fatalities occurred from errors related to misdiagnosis and the level of phenomenon they caused. Even though, an event study provides information to assist with constructing a theoretical probability analysis to indicate the level of incorrect prognosis; investigations gathered from empirical evidence reveals what was certain or impossible to validate occurrences that relates to the quality of care and what caused those occurrences and the reactions from family members. Thus, this study provides evidence that determined whether there was reasons to concentrate on eliminating issues associated with types of bias that would halt continuous research in this field. Furthermore, this research focused on presenting data that provided pertinent information about events, situations, and behaviors with the goal of providing results to understand what caused the occurrences to uncover, interpret, and reflect on solutions while investigating various aspects of those behavior(s). The above information assisted with gathering data that represented and validated the extent of medical errors in each specific category that consist of gender, age, nationality, and/or migration.

The Problem Statement

The problem was medical diagnostic errors, since diagnostic errors account for 17% of preventable incidents and approximately 9% of patients experience major undetected diagnostic errors when they were alive, in addition thousands of patients hospitalized died every year, because of medical errors (Patient Safety Network, 2017). These incidents occurred in categories; such as, medical errors, post-surgical complications, associated infections, in addition landmark patient studies discovered that diagnostic errors are common within the practice (Patient Safety Network, 2017). The information in the preceding article presented a focused view that emphasized improvements can occur by removing areas of bias that are associated with heuristics, in the category of diagnostic impressions that derive from placing undue reliance on expert opinion or total reliance on test results (Patient Safety Network, 2017). Therefore, this information presents evidence to validate that complex interventions are associated with qualitative and/or quantitative issues or occurrences (Higgins et al. 2013). However, the primary purpose for this study was to address the quality of health care, since there was indications there were evasive under-appreciated problems on this topic, which are contributing factors for approximately 10% of patients' death and, as many as 17% of hospitals' adverse events (AE) (McCarthy, 2015; US Institute of Medicine, 2015). In addition, those results indicated a lack of strategic planning when it pertained to quality improvement versus patient safety initiatives, per the most current report during this research from the US Institute of Medicine (McCarthy, 2015; US Institute of Medicine, 2015).

The Purpose for the Study

The purpose for this qualitative research design was to investigate the quality of care in the health-care profession, because of increases in diagnostic and prognosis error rates that caused concerns about behavior(s) that is essential for quality care within the health-care profession, take for example an article in the AARP 2016 Bulletin. The Bulletin indicated the health-care systems might be harming their patients by providing wrong diagnosis, sloppy practices, poor communication, lax hygiene, dismal discharge planning, knowledge gaps, drug blunders, dangerous doctors, outpatient black hole, buried information, clinician burnout, and small talk (National Institute of Health (NIH), 2016). All of which are contributing factors that causes medical and diagnostic errors. Therefore, concerns from this organization erupted in late 1999 when the Institute of Medicine published information that directed concern toward the medical establishment; it estimated that nearly 100,000 hospitalized patients died annually from preventable errors (US Institute of Medicine, 2015). Therefore, reiterating that medical errors was the third-leading cause that attributed to death in the United States, after cancer and heart disease (Abbasi, 2016; Allen, & Pierce, 2016; Daniel, & Makary, 2016; Ginsburg et al. 2016). Furthermore, diagnostic errors has received great attention over the past decade, but the points that was addressed consisted of quantifiable problems associated with health care that pertained to infections, medication errors, and post-surgical complications. Although, these were important issues the argument here was the rising level of error rates in the categories of diagnostic and prognostic medical errors. Thus, concerns continue to arise over quality issues within health-care agencies as they recommended taking a closer look at factors that were associated with human error (AHRQ) Agency for Healthcare Research and Quality, 2016). After 1999 up to 2012, new information indicated that medical errors were the sixth leading cause of death in the United States

(US) and may be as high as 400,000, as the results indicated from a stratified random sample taken from 10 hospitals from January 2002 through 2007 in the state of North Carolina (Harris, & Peeples, 2015). Although, there was suggestions for improving patient safety no significant decrease in medical harm occurred. Therefore, this research validates levels of occurrences and incidents that are associated with diagnostic medical errors to provide a level of strategic approaches to consider for removing barriers for solutions (Harris, & Peeples, 2015). Currently, researchers acknowledge that medical errors should rank as a third leading cause of death, per a study at John Hopkins Medicine (Allen, & Pierce, 2016). In addition, the same research validated that the tracking system of vital statistics indicated important information were outside of the public's eye (Allen, & Pierce, 2016). Based on an analysis of prior research, the Johns Hopkins study estimated that more than 250,000 Americans died each year from medical errors. On the Center for Disease and Control's (CDC's) official list medical errors ranked just behind heart disease and cancer with each taking about 600,000 lives in 2014; thus, those errors were in front of respiratory disease, which caused about 150,000 deaths (Allen, & Pierce, 2016). Additionally, to realize the percentage of medical errors there was an estimation for the U. S. that validated diagnostic errors occurred in 15% of patients who received services from clinics and 12 million adults were affected annually, which led to damages, death or permanent disabilities (Jena, & Khullar, 2016; Jena et al. 2015). Therefore, medical errors was a feasible topic to research primarily within the geographical locations in the U. S.

Research Questions

The research questions provided a constructed to examine behavior(s) and provide data that pertains to decision-making processes. Therefore, using heuristics offers an opportunity to observe behavior(s) that are associated with slow or speedy decision-making processes. In addition, the authors on this topic suggested in certain circumstances diagnostic errors was misconstrued when it pertain to heuristics, because there were indications that content knowledge was the core root of diagnostic performance (Eva, McLaughlin, & Norman, 2014). Therefore, indicating heuristics lies on a casual route between knowledge in comparison to diagnostic errors and success (Eva et al. 2014). Additionally, errors derive from poor communication, lax hygiene, dismal discharge planning, knowledge gap, buried information, clinician burnout, and/or small talk, to name a few (Ginsberg et al. 2016; Daniel, & Makary, 2016). Therefore, presenting characteristics that are associated with self-determination theories, whereas the phenomenon was caused from lack of interest in learning, self-confidence, and/or do not see value in education. Therefore, resulting in lack of teamwork causing an inability to follow instructions, which impairs the ability to identify errors or provide an accurate diagnosis (Jena, & Khullar, 2016). Thus, the research questions addressed the following:

1. Who was present at the onset of the decision-making process?

2. Where did the occurrences occur, and was there referrals made, example, primary care facility, operating room, emergency room, and/or adverse event?

3. When, where, and was return office visits recommended?

These are areas where examining behaviors are essential, because an examination of behavior(s) that address philosophical issue becomes necessary when gathering data that pertain to decision-making processes. The above questions derive from the necessity to focus on onset of symptoms and concerns about addressing the death of thousands of individuals in the United States within the health-care profession with the goal of improving diagnostic processes, because recommendations was made to facilitate effective teamwork during the diagnostic process, educate, and address performances (Cohen, & Michael, 2016). These are important criterion, since having abilities to detect errors in a not so perfect situation can produce positive results, as indicated by the 18% of incorrect diagnoses that was correctly revised while most of the errors went undetected per the article *Reflecting on Diagnostic Errors: Taking a second look is not enough* (Howey, Mazzetti, Monteiro, Norman, Patel, & Sherbino, 2015). However, the overall effects of the study verified a small segment that consisted of a 2% increase for accurate diagnoses and few were changed. In the meantime, those who recognized diagnostic errors corrected the errors. In addition, the results suggested physicians utilize their abilities to self-assess and identify possible errors (Howey et al. 2015). Furthermore, as of 2016 improving diagnostic processes continued receiving great attention within the health-care industry and recommendations was made to facilitate effective teamwork during the diagnostic process to educate and address performances (Cohen, & Michael, 2016).

Theoretical/Conceptual Framework

This construct addresses problematic issues that pertain to accuracy, since suggestions indicated there were certain circumstances when diagnostic errors were misconstrued and was referenced to heuristics, whereas, there was indications that content knowledge was the root of diagnostic performance (Eva, McLaughlin, & Norman, 2014). In the meantime, since there were circumstances when diagnostic errors became misconstrued and content knowledge was the root of diagnostic performance, which required taking a closer look to warn off incidents (Eva et al.

2014). The following information provided the theoretical framework for this study from data associated with slow or speedy decision-making processes that was essential for reducing error rates within the health-care profession. This framework provided the criterion for addressing phenomenon by removing isolated out-liners that are classified as unusual events, whereas, in most instance the errors did not cause harm, although there was continued increase in error rates dating back more than a decade ago, errors continued to rise (Howey et al. 2015). This framework assisted with taking a closer look at data to identify possible causes for increases in error rates (Howey et al. 2015). In addition, it provided criterion necessary to identify technological issues that highlighted high risk factors that might stem from high-technology, high risk procedures, and barriers toward learning (Ginsburg, Levinson, & Yeung, 2016; Eva et al. 2014).

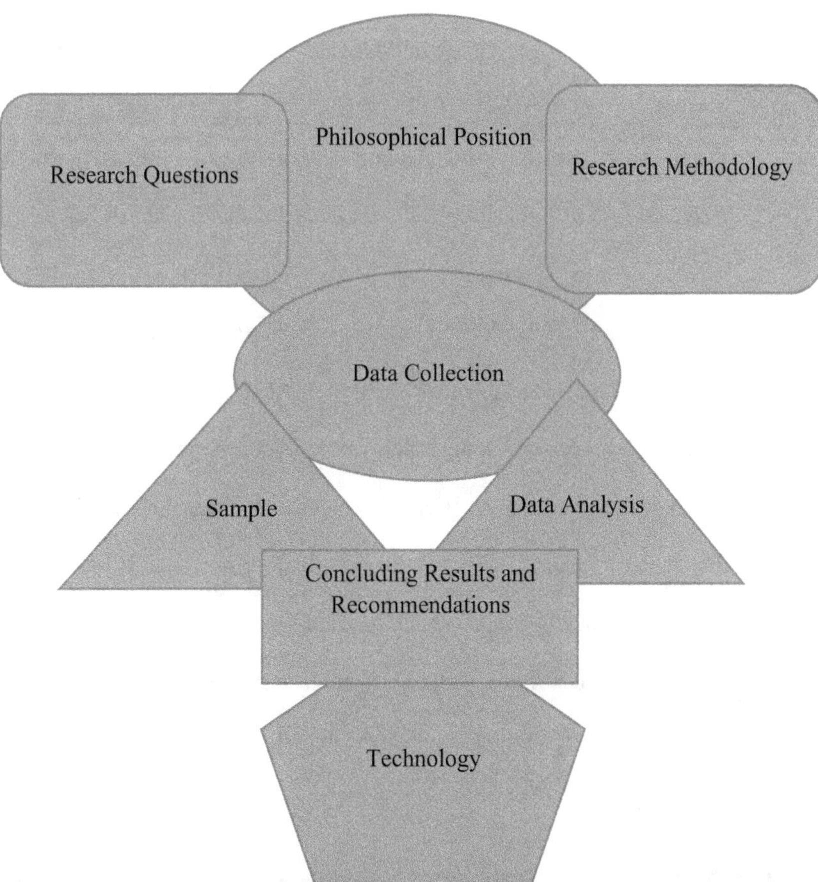

The above framework provided the capability to focus on how independent variables (patients and or technology) influence or cause the dependent variable (health-care professional) to cause phenomenon and increase the pattern above and over the activities of their systems, therefore removing accountability and reference statements, such as, *To Err is Human* (Garber, & Singh, 2015; Priest, 2013)

Nature of the Study

The collected data provided inroads to meaningful information about knowledge, behavior(s), thought(s), and the patients' social network. This process provided data to streamline social determinants that may have an impact on health (National Institute of Health (NIH), 2016). This research provided the foundation that was essential for improving communication, integration, and program coordination; evaluations, and policy-making. In addition, it assisted with implementing strategies to accomplish objectives of each important phenomenon (National Institute of Health (NIH), 2016; National Institute of Health, 2017). Although, physicians, pharmacists, and nurses are trained to work at high proficient levels, as well as, functioning according to their call for action has caused additional concerns when issues was related to high error rates (Eva et al. 2014). This research will benefit the medical profession and assist with improving managerial practices, as well as, contribute to the body of knowledge, therefore, acknowledging the importance of facilitating effective teamwork within the health-care facilities. Primarily, since there was tremendous dependency on electronic communication and many are not effective enough to communicate diagnostic data (Cohen, & Laposata, 2016). The importance for constructing this framework was to formulate a grounded approach, because of the importance of identifying medical errors to correct them. Therefore, the following reminders were designed to reiterate the importance of occurrences during an investigation, because the goal was to determine the level of rare, and adverse events in an emergency department (ED) or Academic Tertiary Care department (Anderson, Chiu, Edlow, Grossman, Klasco, Wolfe, & Wong, 2015). During, this process the design was constructed to collect data on every patient that were referred to a Tertiary Care Academic Medical Facility ED. At the beginning of January 2009 through November 2012, the annual census indicated there were 55,000 patients who were systematically identified with predetermined criteria that was identified by an electronic medical record system (Anderson et al. 2015; Cohen & Laposata, 2016). The information specified the criteria for review that consisted of 72-hour returns to the ED and those admitted on second visits. The patients admitted from ED then transferred to an intensive care unit (ICU) within 24 hours during arrival. It verified if airway management was required and Quality Assurance (QA) committee were involved in solving complaints then the removal of barriers that cause conflicts of interest would be removed, thus physicians who were not involved in the care was assigned to investigate the study (Anderson et al. 2015). The investigation process utilized a structured electronic tool that provided occurrence of error rates and ED. The Beth Israel Deaconess Medical Center Institutional Review Board (IRB) waived the study. Therefore, ensuring the information was worthy of an investigation as it provided data that contributed to the body of knowledge in the field of the health-care industry (Anderson et al. 2015). This provided evidence that focusing on examining the validity structure of qualitative research was essential for providing a distinction between qualitative and quantitative research, because the basic ontological and epistemological assumptions was they are incompatible. Therefore, the concept of validity and reliability should be removed, because most qualitative research have a more moderate viewpoint. This approach required researchers to authenticate their work by referring to qualitative research that was plausible, trustworthy, creditable, and defensible (Gelso, & Silberberg, 2016).

Significance of the Study

The significance of this study was to focus on error rates in the medical profession to contribute to the body of knowledge in the field of business and technology, because the medical institutions consist of various components and when medical errors occur it often causes traumatic experiences that often require counseling for those individuals or family members who experience phenomenon. Therefore, effective communication was required to produce real relationships, in other words, genuine relationship for progressive outcomes (Cheng, Fuertes, Gelso, & Owen, 2013; Gelso, & Silberberg, 2016). This was crucial for establishing goals to eliminate information that has negative influences on relationships and distort the theoretical formulation (Cheng et al. 2013; Gelso, & Silberberg, 2016). As a result this process made allowances to provide and compare trajectory of elements of the relationship in therapy dyads to produce healing and other factors to determine if the relationship between outcomes that was successful versus the dyads that were not successful and resulted in ineffective communication (Cheng et al. 2013). The goal for this research topic was to focus on constructing a theoretical framework that consisted of pertinent information to validate there was inconsistencies within processes. This provided assistance with determining overlaps in therapy for medical profession managers to utilize their strategies to reduce excessive error rates (Cheng et al. 2013). The importance of this section was to validate there is a significant existence between relationships and effective outcomes, because the psychotherapist and clients are viewed as the key variables that attributes to failure or the success of psychotherapy of all theoretical (academia) orientations (Gelso, 2014; Gelso, &

Silberg, 2016). In the meantime, continuous research has provided criterion that needs improvement. Since, prior research has acknowledged that positive relationships had an impact on a patients' outcome and additional research provided strong philosophical theories with imperial data that contributed to the body of knowledge and criterion for theory building to improve performance (Baumann, Gleso, Hill, & Kivlighan, 2016; Cronin, 2014; Gelso, 2014; Gelso, & Silberg, 2016).

Definition of Key Terms

Although, the information under this subheading is pertaining to years prior to 2012 it provides information to validate how medical errors and fatal incident occurs. Take for instance, what occurred from 2000 through 2007 when there were an inaccurately diagnose multi-drug resistant pathogens that rapidly spread, because of greater networking it caused infections to spread quicker than in previous years (Jena, & Khullar, 2016). This article concentrated on prognostic errors instead of primarily diagnostic errors and the results from this study focused on the importance of acknowledging there are variances in outcome due to health conditions, which was an important issue that generated great concern from the Institute of Medicine, during 2015 (Jena, & Khullar, 2016). In other words, it was important to identify flaws to determine how often diagnoses was inaccurate and how often the delivery system fails. This systemic strategy assisted with locating flaws that identified causes that pertain to measurements and/or education (Jena, & Khullar, 2016). Therefore, factors to consider that pertain to measurements and/or education consisted of error, bias, thinking, decision-making, and meta-cognition, which relates to the research questions (Brügger, & Kretzchmar, 2015; Hamilton & Trimble, 2016). This was important since diagnostic errors are the same as incorrect diagnoses of medication, because the only difference was the errors occur due to lack of adequate prescription or wrong medication (Daniel, & Makay, 2016; Anderson et al. 2015). Researching information that pertains to phenomenological methods provides a description of the phenomenon that relates to everyday experiences that was associated with the problems to provide information that is essential for formatting the overall structure. This process required focusing on ethnography and the grounded theories for incorporating hermeneutics during the research process to provide relationships that focused on the following key terms:

1. **Adverse Events** – Life threatening occurrences caused by diagnostic errors classified as an untoward medical occurrence in a patient or clinician; when a pharmaceutical product does not necessarily have a causal relationship with that treatment (Anderson et al. 2015).

2. **Analyst Triangulation** - Refers to analyst of multiple sources to review findings to illuminate blind spots when focusing on an interpretive analysis (Eva et al. 2014).

3. **Bias** - Prejudices made by experts in any field against a person, group, or person by comparing others in an unfair manner (Hamilton, & Trimble, 2016).

4. **Conflicts** – Consist of clashes, incompatibility, dissension, and/or serious disagreements (Garber, & Singh, 2015; Jena et al. 2015).

5. **Diagnostic Medical Errors** – Are mistakes omitted by health-care professionals that result in harm to the patient (Howey et al. 2015; McCarthy, 2015).

6. **Errors** - The state of being wrong, a mistake (Hamilton, & Trimble, 2016).

7. Hermeneutics - Is a study of human behavior and social institutions in the categories of the bible, theology, and/or philosophy (Eva et al. 2014).

8. Iatrogenic damage - Is a state of illness or an adverse effect from the result of medical treatment (Daniel & Makary, 2016).

9. Misclassification - Placed in a wrong category (Jena et al. 2015).

10. Misconstrue - Misunderstanding of meaning; to misinterpret (Garber, & Singh, 2015; Jena et al. 2015).

11. Misdiagnoses - Is a diagnosis that is mistaken for another condition (Howey et al. 2015; Mascherek, & Schwappach, 2016).

12. Presentism – A present day point of views; modern medical care (Hamilton, & Trimble, 2016).

13. Prognosis – A prediction made by experts in any field about a recovery or illness (Jena, et al. 2016).

14. Pulmonary Embolism - Occurs when there is a blockage in one artery of the lungs. It occurs when a piece of a blood clot located somewhere else in the body breaks off and travels through the blood stream and inters into an artery that supply the lung (Jena, & Khullar, & 2015).

15. Qualitative data - Information not based on numbers, but is descriptive and the categories can be physical traits, gender, or color (Berg et al. 2016).

Research Method

The research method consists of utilizing the phenomenological method to provide a description of the phenomenon that relates to experiences for determining causes associated with each occurrence to streamline the results to events that cause phenomenon, such as everyday experiences that relates to pain, trauma, and other issues that are associated with well-being (Giorgi, 2013). This approach provided percentages that highlighted areas that need improvement and to formulate data in a structured pattern for guidance, during this research process. Therefore, providing and ensuring the information about the nature of occurrences and incidents was data that validated the grounded theory that related to diagnostic medical errors within the health-care profession. The beginning process began with ethnography, which required gathering information to elaborate on activities of specific groups, as well as, interaction, and communication between group members as it relates to phenomenological research method (Giorgi, 2013). This guaranteed the information validated medical errors presents challenging problems by verifying there was little improvement on the level of misdiagnosed cases. Furthermore, this process assisted with incorporating various aspects of hermeneutics to provide insight from online references that provided a starting point, in terms of where the data began up to the end of conducting this research on the topic of medical errors to provide reasons for actions and phrases.

Collaboration during the research process occurred during the observation process by utilizing the material retrieved from online scholarly, *Academic Journals*, empirical evidence, *Medical Journals*, peered review, news articles, and university libraries sources. The goal for this qualitative research method was to provide autonomy that provided philological historical insight and serve as a guideline to focus on the concept *To Err is Human* (Garber, & Singh, 2015). Since, concepts has the tendency to creep into society as they gasp a hold on ideas they spread throughout cultures and cause conflicts, which provides evident that conflicts do occur, because of communicating errors. Therefore, it was beneficial to interpret the correct meaning from information that comes from research data that involves health-care facilities with the primary goal of providing justice for humans by developing theories that provide evidence for improving qualitative measures within health-care systems. This process requires providing critical distinction between information that transcend from empirical evidence (Giorgi, 2013). The importance of the hermeneutic approach was to provide an understanding of the nature of errors and various conflicting views to zero in on the quality of service and the individual's ability to adhere to instructions. Therefore, searching for information for open-end question was a reasonable approach for exploratory data collection that was unrestricted, since statistical data was not necessary to validate data in qualitative research to formulate the findings. This process provided answers to who, what, when, and how incidents occurred to receive accurate data and conclusions. The benefit of utilizing the qualitative approach drew attention toward the urgency of reducing diagnostic error occurrences. This was important since there were committees who created reports and emphasize the importance of testing selections to interpret results (Cohen, & Laposata, 2016). The purpose for this approach removed areas that cause guessing, although most treating physicians do not want to acknowledge diagnostic errors (Cohen, & Laposata, 2016).

Operational Definition of Variables

Construct/Variable 1. The variables focused on how occurrences occurred and how incidents and/or occurrence affected the targeted group or subject. This process assisted with addressing the individuals' perspective on how interactions between the medical professional and patient derived at the specific diagnoses. Data collection varies from retrieval of archival sources that consist of the internet and/or geographical locations where age had a bearing on error rates or there was no companion to assist with delivering instructions, survey information derived from previous surveys constructed from prior and current research for summing or averaging responses from archival information.

Construct/Variable 2. Under the descriptive variable, it focused on descriptions and the grounded theory to provide an understanding of social and/or psychological processes that characterize situations and events. In addition, information under this construct provided historical data for a systematic method for collecting data from past and current information for the percentage of medical errors under the above categories listed in the category of *construct/variable 1*. This process highlighted trends of consistent and inconsistent behavior(s) that have influence on the decision-making process as these behavior(s) lead up to events and/or occurrences with the goal of reducing excessive error rates. Therefore, constructing a flow chart that served as a guideline assisted with gathering pertinent information for consistency and containment of information for accomplishing the following:

1. Maintaining structure

2. Provide consistent data

3. Gather multiple material from different sources

4. Avoid generalizing

5. The primary goal was to construct data to reduce medical error rates and provide a contribution to the body of knowledge

Measurement

This qualitative study, concentrates on constructs, such as, data collection from observation of prior research of scholarly, empirical, peer reviewed articles; medical journals, and education materials that provides pertinent information on diagnostic medical error for delivery toward the purpose of this study. The purpose for gathering material on medical errors was to determine whether the errors could be systematic. In addition, to eliminating breakdown in communication and individualized errors, or if they were attributed to high-risk populations that consisted of men and the elderly who may require more physical examinations to decrease medical errors and/or coordination of efforts to improve communication among residents who was treating the same patient (Arnold et al. 2013; Harris, & Peeples, 2015). Therefore, the goal was to provide data for constructing a comparative research design that provided data from the period of five years or less (Harris, & Peeples, 2015).

The results from this qualitative approach was for providing information to consider from previous studies that validate complex intervention that was associated with qualitative issues or occurrences (Higgins et al. 2013). In addition, the goal was to gather qualitative data in a cross-language context for synthesizing evidence that caused complex intervention. Therefore, when focusing on the decision-making processes, it provided measures for qualitative approaches to address the research problem. This eliminated the necessity to review different research designs to arrive at an adequate conclusion. The following was an excellent example, because prior research in 2012 provided a two-way workshop that were held in Canada to construct measures for intervening to reduce the number of medical errors, which has been ineffective during the last decade. Therefore, by developing a standard meta-analysis that provided a comparison between previous and current research the goal was to identify and provide statistical measurements to share from each study that provided the effected size. The results assisted with determining the sample size to investigate what was important for determining quality of health care; although, it was widely assumed that medical errors follow a Gaussian distribution, whereas they may follow a Power Rule distribution (Higgins et al. 2013). Therefore, information presented in the research provided evidence in favor of a Power Rule distribution for medical errors and then examined the consequences of such a distribution. Since, the distribution of medical errors had real-world implications, further research was necessary to determine whether medical errors follow a Gaussian or Power Rule distribution. In the meantime, there was little evidence that there was reform in this area, because data from both sides of the Atlantic suggested that despite numerous interventions to improve the quality of health care the last decade indicated that the quality of care was deteriorating despite health-care providers receiving quality care training (Higgins et al. 2013). The conclusion indicated further research was necessary to contribute to the body of knowledge.

Summary

The above information validated diagnostic errors received a great amount of attention over the past decades and the criteria consisted of errors that were quantified problems in health care, such as infections, medication errors, and post-surgical complications (AHRQ Agency for Healthcare Research and Quality, 2016). Although, those errors are just as important as qualified problems this research approach addressed the quality of health care to ensure patient safety, however a small amount of information has addressed the frequent usage of heuristics. In other words, short cuts to remove many biases that are associated with availability or anchoring biases (AHRQ, 2016). Further, research provided information to determine if levels of human errors are still on the rise, because when errors occur to the extent of those listed above, they have an impact on professional services when incidents do not improve and they cause complexities in the health-care industry. Thus, the situation draws critical concerns and create phenomenon, since diagnostic errors increase clinical stress and excessive financial burdens on the institutions that are involved and their patients (Jena et al. 2015). This was an area where reasoning abilities are crucial, since it plays a role in decision-making processes. It was important to seek results, because occurrences often are related the staffs' well-being when it related to burnout (Hall, Johnson, O'Conner, Tsipa, &Watt, 2016). Furthermore, there was evidence from 16 out of 27 studies that validated well-being had a significant correlation between poor well-being and inadequate patient safety (Hall et al. 2016). This was another important issue to consider, since employees within the medical facilities and their patients are associating with experiences, such as, anxiety and/or depression levels; likewise, many of the health-care professionals are also experiencing the above characteristics and/or display forms of mannerism that produce negative and/or positive results. Therefore, utilizing statistical data can provide information for specified criteria to evaluate (Bennett et al. 2014; Hall et al. 2016).

Take for example, what occurred in New Zealand there was one nurse practitioner registered in 2002, and in the early portion of 2012, 100 nurse practitioners were registered (Boyd, Gagan, Williams, & Wysocki, 2014; Pirret, 2016). Under the title of nurse practitioner, they receive protection under their title, because they earned their master's degree and New Zealand allows them to independently practice without supervision of a physician (Pirret, 2016). This was an important factor to take into consideration, since nurse practitioners and resident doctors possess diagnostic reasoning that provide similar outcome for patients; however, it was important to remember that medical doctors (MD) holds the highest credentials (LaGrow, Neville, & Pirret, 2015; Pirret, 2016). Therefore, accurate collection of data assessments that are relevant to a case is essential, because it provides the capability to integrate data from stored knowledge to derive at adequate conclusions, however cognitive resources can become overloaded and cause error in diagnoses (Eva, McLaughlin, & Norman, 2014; Hall et al. 2016; Pirret, 2016). In the meantime, there were no positive results noted in a case study that pertained to a dermatologist who after completing skin biopsies on 2 of his patients realized when beginning the 3rd procedure the instrument was not sterilized nor were any of the trays (Ginsburg, Levinson, & Yeung, 2016). Although, the health-care professional knew the risk of infections from unsterilized equipment were low, but blood-borne pathogens can transmit infectious diseases, such as, hepatitis and HIV transmitted diseases, it resulted in the professional experiencing a dilemma that could have caused bias in decision-making. Therefore, presenting cause for conflict in ethical decision-making, since patients must be notified about the incident (Ginsburg et al. 2016). The most important information to take away from this experience was that guidelines are established to disclose medical errors, therefore it does require following guidelines to highlight diagnostic errors (Arnold et al. 2013; Ginsburg et al. 2016).

Chapter 2: Literature Review

This research paper was to reiterate the importance of realizing life provides a tremendous amount of learning experience and it was an organization/business' responsibility to accept new and additional materials that coincide with specific subject matters, and in this case the medical profession, because this literature review

provides information for improvement purposes. The reasons are because prior to the

year of 2012, research has validated how and why medical errors occur by

acknowledging there were inaccuracies when diagnosing multi-drug pathogens and as

greater networking occurred, it caused infections to spread rapidly (Jena, & Khullar,

2016). Therefore, this information verified communication breakdown, poor

judgment, diagnostic errors, and inadequate skills can result in direct harm or death of

a patient, since these acts are the result of failure to execute or inadequate planning

medical errors can occur on a system level or from an individuals' action (Daniel, &

Makary, 2016; Diagnostic Errors/AHRQ Patient Safety Network, 2017). This

required preventing preventable lethal events that becomes complex and produce

phenomenon was essential (Daniel, & Makary, 2016). Per the article that focused on

how big was the problem, there was information dated back as far as 1984 from a

Harvard study, which argued that the estimation in the study were low, because 78%

rather than 51% of the cases were iatrogenic deaths that were preventable (Daniel, &

Makary, 2016). In order, to elaborate further iatrogenic damage was a state of illness

or an adverse effect from the result of medical treatment and it was the third major

cause of death in the US following cancer and heart disease (Daniel, & Makary,

2016). Therefore, it was important to ensure health-care practices are not rooted deep

in phenomenology, which consist of continental philosophical tradition that stem from

Husserl (1859-1938) who was a German mathematician, as well as, logician (Priest,

2013). This was because when it pertains to *To Err is Human* attention was directed

to Husseri who believed all knowledge is a product of experience that pertain to an

abstract concept, physical object, or a mood (Priest, 2013). To emphasize the

importance of this problem the Institute of Medicine reiterated the importance of maintaining quality health care, by providing adequate information to remove blind spots, since delays and/or inaccurate information has an impact on quality care. This article identified area that cause diagnostic errors, which consist of failure to explain the patients' problem(s) with accuracy and having the ability to communicate the report to emphasize the urgency of the problem(s) that must be addressed (Hamilton & Trimble, 2016; US Institute of Medicine, 2015). The importance of this approach was to provide a leeway to address challenging situations, which can eliminate most diagnostic errors with the goal of improving error rates; since this process will benefit families, researchers, patients, health-care professionals, health-care organization, and policy makers as updated data contributes to the body of knowledge (Sarma, 2015; US Institute of Medicine, 2015). Examining behavior(s) becomes necessary when providing data that pertain to decision-making processes. Furthermore, there were authors who suggest using heuristics, because it offers an opportunity for observing behavior(s) that are associated with slow or speedy decision-making processes (Eva, McLaughlin, & Norman, 2014). In the meantime, when it pertained to heuristics in circumstances diagnostic errors were misconstrued, therefore indicating that content knowledge was the root of diagnostic performance. Thus, the authors' recommendations suggested heuristics lies on a casual route between knowledge in comparison to diagnostic error or success. Thus, it requires designing research methods for qualitative data that is void of the design of quantitative research methods to provide data to validate the findings (Sarma, 2015). This provided the opportunity to develop data with shared leadership management teams to conduct a study that investigates excessive levels of misdiagnosed cases to determine if the percentage of these cases have decreased or increased over the last few years. This was important since there was information that verified nurse practitioners serves as a valuable contributor for the health-care profession. As a result this comparative research design validated that their reasoning abilities compares to that of medical doctors when confronted with managing complex cases, meanwhile, it was important to remember medical doctors (MD) holds the highest credentials in their profession (LaGrow et al. 2015). Furthermore, additional information from another study indicated medical related expenses have totaled 60% of bankruptcies and ¾ of those bankruptcies happen to those patients with health insurance (Affordable Care Act Summary, 2014). The data from this investigation provided a voice for patients, clients, and it improved communication for those who receive services in agencies, such as hospitals or clinics. However, the argument here was the challenges that occur when it pertains to medical errors; there was little emphases placed on occurrences and individual thoughts and the impact those thoughts had on reasoning and good decision-making strategies that assisted with focusing on key factors to minimize errors (Hamilton & Trimble, 2016). Other areas of concerns derive from the death of thousands individuals in the United States (US) within the health-care profession. Therefore, improving diagnostic processes was receiving great attention in the health-care field and recommendations were made to facilitate effective teamwork during the diagnostic process, educate, address performances, technological support must coincide with patient diagnoses, and suggestion were made to dedicate funding for research to ensure each error was identified and addressed (Cohen & Laposata, 2016; Cohen & Michael, 2016). Since, patients are not necessarily the solution when it comes to errors in health-care facilities, such as, primary care due to ineffective communication from lack of knowledge on medical topics; therefore, it were essential that communication was clear and concise to identify challenging health conditions. Although, quantified problems are just as important as qualified problems and minimum attention addressed levels of quality within the health-care profession, therefore, the urgency to monitor and improve the level of diagnostic error rates was increasing (AHRQ, 2016). However, there are important issues that are associated with diagnostic and prognostic medical errors when it comes to quality; because as the world strives to become as one by integrating Christian living, it requires providing measures for national, and international challenges that can cause conflicts, bias, and have an impact on improving the quality of care (Brügger, & Kretzschmar, 2015).

The above information was important, since diagnostic errors account for 17% of preventable errors in patients hospitalized and approximately 9% of patients experience major undetected diagnostic errors while patients were alive, per Harvard Medical Practice study; in addition, thousands of patients died every year, because of diagnostic errors (Patient Safety Network, 2016). In addition, long term care was on the rise and a major error in this category was failure to communicate, which leads to unnecessary hospitalizations for conditions that require long-term care situations (Carrington, & Renz, 2016; Goodman, Kuo, & Raji, 2013). Concerns grew in late1999, when the Institute of Medicine published information that directed attention toward the medical establishment and provided an estimation that nearly 100,000 hospitalized patients die annually from preventable error (Abbasi, 2016) and the perspective for this research was to focus on understanding behaviors that can have an impact on diagnostic and prognostic medical error rates. This information validated that medical errors was the third-leading cause for death in the United States, after cancer and heart disease. Furthermore, the information provided in the AARP Bulletin coincides with previous research, because it reiterated the importance of reducing medial errors, although it was human to make mistakes. Additional information validates 90,000 deaths was preventable that involved hospital acquired infections (Abbasi, 2016). The above information provides important facts to consider, because the primary purpose of health-care providers was to strive toward providing quality care and a just culture that was willing to contribute to the body knowledge with the goal of reducing and/or eliminating error rates in the health-care industry (Arnold, et al. 2013). The data from this study was to identify problems that are associated with medical errors and answer the questions that pertain to inefficiencies, bias, and/or lack of communication. Therefore, verifying there are positive relationships that are associated with health-care team members' communication skills, along with a patient's capacity to adhere to medical recommendations that will assist with improving managing medical errors and procedures. These are a few issues at the forefront of diagnostic errors, therefore, it was crucial to understand how to detect the system-based intervention plans at the beginning process that overlap errors during onset of diagnosis and prognosis (Garber, & Singh, 2015). However, there are circumstances when errors occur that has an impact on business ethics, because there are many religious denominations whose beliefs have an impact on the quality of health care that relates to their religious beliefs (Brügger, & Kretzschmar, 2015). Therefore, integrating Christian living and management toward national and international challenges can pose conflict of interest if diagnostic measurements are not handled appropriate and accurately (Brügger, & Kretzschmar, 2015). Thus, (Brügger, & Kretzschmar, 2015) researched how Christian living and international management practice can integrate, to remove conflict of interest. This was an important criterion, since within some Christian-theological approaches to business ethics there are certain management practitioners who practice separation between work and faith (Brügger, & Kretzschmar, 2015). To reiterate the importance of this main facet of ethical standard in business, Nils Ole Oerman, 2007, argued that in the business enterprise it was the main challenge of business (Brügger, & Kretzschmar, 2015). Empirical evidence exposed a paradox as it revealed Christian living, including some managers separate work from faith, because of reducing faith to application of principles that was ethical, therefore, reducing criterion that pertains to ethics to a limiting-practice function (Brügger, & Kretzschmar, 2015). Furthermore, the data indicated that separation between managerial practice and faith was questionable. The results indicated from the empirical analysis there was no solution to those problems that caused phenomenon between decision-making based on the principles outlined for separation between faith and work (Brügger, & Kretzschmar, 2015). Nevertheless, there was data that revealed practical problems associated with issues caused by separations, such as, conflicts that arouse, because of those who presented one's own views as economic truth, because they failed to state assumptions associated and underpinned those views (Brügger, & Kretzschmar, 2015). The preceding information provided attributes that formulate faith based on beliefs about realities that influence business practice and the results indicates the problems when there are assumptions about radical gaps between practice and faith; because assumptions correspond with inadequacies of the practices that are associated with gaps that relates to gaps within the theoretical faith-practices (Brügger, & Kretzschmar, 2015). This topic was not only apparent in international management, since it does appear in business strategies and/or cooperation's nationally. Other segments within the health-care system that require quality care are nursing homes, because nursing home care varies greatly (Goodman, Kuo, & Raji, 2013). On this topic, information from a study conducted in nursing homes in Texas during 2006-2008 focused on 12,249 newly admitted patients to long-term care and identified by Medicare Claims to a minimum data set of 100%

(Goodman et al. 2013). The process provided measures of care over six months and

the claims potentially avoidable were over a period of 6-28 months. The conclusion

validated the efforts the providers devoted to nursing homes were associated with

avoidable risk to the emergency department (ED) and hospitalizations, primarily

because of unavailable primary care providers within their facilities (Goodman et al.

2013). According, to experts' mental health has been a seriously neglected category

that was overlooked, primarily because of different characteristics that are composed

of attributes of patients, treatment, and setting (Mascherek, & Schwappach, 2016).

Therefore, a study provided constructs to combine knowledge from research in the

field to provide existing initiatives and projects that would define priorities for patient

safety, in the category of mental health-care in Switzerland (Mascherek, &

Schwappach, 2016). The design for this study was a modified Delphi questionnaire, a

semi structured questionnaire, and two around table questionnaire to gauge experts'

opinion that pertain to priorities in patient safety in Switzerland's mental health care

between May 2015 and October 2015 (Mascherek, & Schwappach, 2016). The

results provided nine pathways that consisted of medication errors, diagnostic errors,

non-drug errors, treatment errors, errors related to aggressive management against self

and others, communication errors, errors that pertain to suicidal tendencies in patients,

structural errors, and errors at interfaces of care where patients and organizations met

and/or interact (Mascherek, & Schwappach, 2016). The conclusion of the study

provided evidence that patient safety was important to provide quality care in the

mental health category, per experts, because diagnostic errors were on top of the

priority list (Mascherek, & Schwappach, 2016). Errors are not uncommon, therefore

exploring categories that may have an impact on the decision-making processes for individuals who suffer from mental conditions, such as, ADHD and other similar conditions that cause deficits in rational reasoning is essential. Primarily, since these could cause an impact on cognitive abilities, effect social rule, and memory integration (Brunamonti, Costanzo, Ferraina, Mammi, Menghini, Pani, Rufini, Veneziani, & Vicari, 2017; Preston, & Schlichting, 2015). These are a few issues at the forefront of diagnostic errors, therefore, it was crucial to understand how to detect the systems-based intervention plans at the beginning process that overlap the errors during onset of diagnosis and prognosis, since sharing information trigger reactivation of previous learned experience (Brunamonti et al. 2017; Dominick, Preston, & Zeithamova, 2012; Garber, & Singh, 2015). In order, to understand children with attention deficit hyper activity disorder (ADHD) there were an observational study to validate the children were impaired when they performed inferential reasoning problems to derive at a conclusion, because there was a delay or difficulty in managing unified representation of ordered items (Brunamonti et al. 2017). Behaviors are important to understand, because reflecting on the past provides an understanding about current experiences and predictions that pertain to future occurrences (Dominick et al. 2012). Therefore, it was essential to understand how memories can be successful to generate actions or future judgments, because it was the criteria for relating information during multiple episodes (Dominick et al. 2012). The study, also, provided clarity by providing a deeper understanding to elaborated on how past experiences provided the ability to learn current information (Dominick et al. 2012). The goal for revealing this information improved behaviors and mediated integration enables inference across experiences (Dominick et al. 2012; Preston, & Schlichting, 2015). Meanwhile, reflecting on the Institutional Review Board (IRB), since they serve as a guideline to ensure protection for all human subjects by ensuring the highest ethic and scientific standards are in adherence to ethical principles outlined in the Belmont report will serve as a protection (National Institute of Environmental Health Sciences, 2017). Furthermore, misdiagnosis was one of the phenomenon that was research worthy when it pertained to conflict management, which can become contributing factors on top of the list causes for medical malpractice payout, per a report from the 2015 Institute of medicine (Busch, 2016; US Institute of Medicine, 2015). Therefore, the goal was to provide an understanding to eliminate the notion to "do as you please," because medial errors in most circumstances cause harm (Gapp, & Stewart, 2017). There was value added when qualitative research investigated a topic for crystallizing for understanding world surroundings, as it adds vigor for research and the researchers' position (Brunamonti et al, 2017; Gapp, & Stewart, 2017). This process provided alchemy for deeper understanding about phenomenon by understanding occurrences from prior literature and the value of continuous research on this topic, since conflict management and cultural differences can influence medical practices (Busch, 2016; Gapp, & Stewart, 2017). This was an excellent process to focus on when initiating solutions that are associated with blind spots to highlight assumptions that can be corrected (Busch, 2016; Gapp, & Stewart, 2017). Cultural theories are areas that require reiterating the importance of questioning intercultural mediation, because of limited research or questioning on conflicting managerial practices. Therefore, the author indicated that in multi-factor ways there are articles designed that consider how cultural relativist attitudes may stem from intercultural research (Busch, 2016). As a result, the author implied that mediation manageable cases designed from procedures that involve initiating designs for approaching conflict management was research worthy (Busch,

2016). These are very important pointers to consider when research data was applicable to diagnostic medical errors.

Purpose of the Study

There are numerous theories that can provide a contribution to analyze causes for excessive error rates in the medical profession. Consequently, in multi-facet ways there are articles that provide relativist attitudes that derive from intercultural research (Busch, 2016). The results from this type of research provided the capability to utilize the quality management system (QMS) that covered vase areas, since developing a framework, such as, this would provide information for a framework to identify measures for developing flexible data for clinical research (Bergamo et al. 2016). The goal was to provide clarity for regulators on expectations in a clinical framework to support organizations for evaluation purposes, tools, and resources (Bergamo et al. 2016). However, the primary purpose for this qualitative study was to provide comparative data to determine if there was a reduction in medical errors so it highlights areas in need of improvement. These concerns are important, because providing quality care requires initiating measures that benefits both patients and clinicians to minimize errors and ensure they are at a minimum. Therefore, providing strategies that consist of patient-reported out measures (PROMS) are essential (Feeny, & Santana, 2014). The information in this literature review focuses on patient safety, patient's families, and the importance of integrity in the health-care profession. The research was to reiterate the importance of adequate and sufficient training, since error rates draws attention to quantified and qualitative problems. In addition, prior evidence indicates complex intervention may be associated with qualitative and/or quantitative issues or occurrences, however, utilizing the qualitative approach provided the best framework to narrow down cause and effects and support findings that relate memory and relational network through retrieval-mediated learning (Higgins et al. 2013; Dominick et al. 2012). Furthermore, the information from this qualitative approach verified most human errors in health care originates from biases and cognitive errors that can be corrected (Bihari et al. 2017). This information provides evidence that medical errors occurred during decision-making processes, as data verified that cognitive errors consisted of (90%), anchoring (75.7%), and premature closure (PC) (78.6%); therefore, validating these are areas in need of improvement (Bihari et al. 2017). In addition, the information presented in the study demonstrated that medical errors was most when it pertains to preventable clinical decision-making, since most of the complaints were about emergency physicians and delayed or missed diagnoses (Bihari et al. 2017). Unfortunately, the study presented no evidence that indicated any changes in prevalence during various cognitive errors. The limitations in this study indicated internal consistency were poor and over confidence level were low, although the basic training focused on teamwork (Bihari et al. 2017). There are additional studies that addressed the quality of health care, since current research indicates there are still an evasive under-appreciated problem on this topic this was a research worthy problem, which are contributing factors for approximately 10% of patients' death and, as many as 17% of hospitals' adverse events (AE) (McCarthy, 2015; US Institute of Medicine, 2015). Further research on this topic indicated a lack of strategic planning when it pertains to quality improvement versus patient safety initiatives, per the most current report from the US Institute of Medicine (McCarthy, 2015; US Institute of Medicine, 2015). In the meantime, the purpose for this study was to remain focus and reiterate the importance of noticing clinical changes by ensuring thorough communication was available as the data on this topic validated (Carrington & Renz, 2016). This process verified that not only verbal communication, but also written communication was essential to ensure continuous improvement within health-care (Carrington, & Renz, 2016). The information provided data that focused on preventing errors by double checking beginning primarily with the front-line practitioners. This was because alternate views attributes to weaknesses when double-checking and different views occur when deciding to double check (Chreim, Forster, & Hewitt, 2016). To improve alternate views, require a dedicated environment, thoroughness, and training; along with reiterating the importance of questioning, since there are limitations to processes, therefore strengthening the ubiquitous of the practice, because it was rarely challenged (Chreim et al. 2016).

Adequate information was essential for improving error rates in the area of medical imaging, because it had posed some issues that pertain to image registration and was the most important task for an effective medical image analysis, as well as, the most critical step for several clinical applications (Alam et al. 2017). The benefits of medical imaging techniques have led to the advancement in computer-assisted surgery (CAS) and radiotherapy (Alam et al. 2017). The purpose for utilizing this technique provides benefits for fast recovery, which assists clinician with qualitative diagnosis to resect the tumor from the information on the image (Alam et al. 2017). Medical imaging was critical for carrying out accurate diagnosis and provides assurance of successful treatment; medical imaging registration entails aligning images to provide a comparison between the patient with normal condition and those with different conditions. Additionally, there are several different types imaging modalities, but each extract different types of information and have their own features for extracting different types of information, since imaging modalities have their own features to extract different information designed for human organs. The importance of this information was to reiterate that accuracy was essential; because describing techniques and familiarity with image registration background knowledge for medical image registration assists with presenting the main issues. Primarily those that cause challenges where possible solutions can be determined for image registration to provide guidelines that are helpful for developing new techniques (Alam et al. 2017).

The authors of this researched issue focused on high morbidity and mortality caused by Lower Respiratory Tract Infection (LRTI) in elderly patients to validate how delay in treatment can cause exacerbation of infections. Therefore, requiring identifying its cause, because there are several causes for the infection and it was important for determining if the condition was associated with pneumonia (Durmaz, Ergun, Ertugrul, Kalem, & Ozdemir, 2017). The means age in this research topic was 73.3 years and each patient that was intubated were hospitalized for more than ten days with trauma, cardiac arrest, pulmonary disease, and other condition, which was a challenge for determining if a patient had pneumonia (Durmaz, et al. 2017). Since, patients in an Intensive Care Unit (ICU) had conditions that consist of multi-morbidities more than one parameter was required and additional studies can validate the value of the test that determine the extent of the infection (Durmaz et al. 2017). Although, extensive research examined the cause of diagnostic errors at individual clinician levels to determine how individuals process information was valuable the clinicians frequently use heuristics primarily with patients who had common symptoms (Diagnostic Errors/AHRQPatient Safety Network, 1017). However, incorrect application of heuristics attributes to cognitive bias, such as, diagnoses based on experiences with past cases, premature closure despite subsequent information, focusing on subtle cues that cause errors when diagnosing, and bias that lead to developing blind obedience, which was a major contributor for diagnostic medical errors (Diagnostic Errors/AHRQ Patient safety Network, 2017). The goal for this research was to unravel causes for diagnostic medical errors, in order to provide data to remove future occurrences toward patients who undergo surgery on wrong body parts, incorrect procedures, or procedures intended for another person (Diagnostic Errors/AHRQ Patient Safety Network, 2017).

Theoretical conceptual framework

This qualitative study, concentrate on constructs, such as, data collection from observation of prior research of scholarly, empirical, peer reviewed articles; medical journals, and education materials that provide pertinent information on diagnostic medical error for delivery toward the purpose of this study (Kulkarni, 2016). The purpose for gathering material on medical errors was to determine whether the errors could be systematic or due to breakdown in communication and not individualized errors. Therefore, highlighting high-risk populations that consist of men and the elderly who may require more physical examinations to decrease medical errors and/or coordination of efforts to improve communication among residents who are treating the same patient (Harris, & Peeples, 2015; Arnold et al. 2013). This resulted in constructing a comparative research design that provided data from the period of five years or less (Harris, & Peeples, 2015). The results from this qualitative approach provide information to consider from previous and current studies to validate complex intervention may be associated with qualitative issues or occurrences (Higgins et al. 2013). Additionally, when focusing on the theoretical framework for nursing educators the study indicated challenges were present when it pertained to handling complex medical care in real life situations according to the study designed to determine the ability to make clinical judgment. In this situation, the authors constructed high-fidelity simulation (HFS) to assess student nurses to determine their teams' abilities to judge by noticing, interpreting, and responding to complex area situations (Hallin, Bäckström, Häggström, & Kristiansen, 2016). The results indicated low clinical judgment for students in their first meeting; although they were in the developing and beginning stages the study validates further research was necessary to focus on health-care experience, age, and assistant nurse degrees, since they were rated second under the categories of decision making, problem solving, clinical judgment, and reasoning (Hallin et al. 2016). These are valuable contributing factors to consider for providing information that pertains to interpretations or conclusion about concerns, health problems, and patients' needs, which are the basis for decision-making to modify approaches or provide provision for new responses with the goal of minimizing errors (Hallin et al. 2016). Therefore, the method for this study remained focused on misdiagnosed cases and qualitative information, since quality was a major concern. In addition, the study focuses on presenting information to understand what caused the occurrences for uncovering, interpreting, and reflecting on solutions while investigating various aspects of behavior(s) that are contributing factors for medical errors. The data presents validation of the extent of medical errors in each specific category, such as, gender, age, nationality, and/or migration. This provided further evidence that there was a lack of strategic planning when it pertained to quality improvement versus patient safety initiatives, per the most current report from the US Institute of Medicine (US Institute of Medicine, 2015; McCarthy, 2015). Based on an analysis from John Hopkins previous research an estimation of more than 250,000 Americans die each year from medical errors and on the Center for Disease and Controls (CDCs) official list medical errors rank behind heart disease and cancer with each taking about 600,000 lives in 2014 (Allen, & Pierce, 2016). Furthermore, those errors were in front of respiratory disease, which caused about 150,000 deaths (Allen, & Pierce, 2016).

The above subheading provides a construct to address problematic issues that pertain to accuracy, since there was an indication that in certain circumstances when diagnostic errors are misconstrued the errors were reference to heuristics, which provided indications that content knowledge was the root of diagnostic performances (Eva et al. 2014). Therefore, providing reliable data to replicate was necessary so others can benefit from the results. Additionally, the information provided a distinct starting points from here to there and the criterion assists with answering the questions that pertain to how and why an incident occurred (Ardhendu, 2014). The following information provided the theoretical framework for this study by providing data associated with slow or speedy decision-making processes that are essential for reducing error rates within the health-care profession. This framework provides criterion for addressing phenomenon and taking a closer look at data to identify possible causes that increase error rates.

Research Questions

The research questions focused on patient safety throughout the medical profession, since there were many areas in the health-care profession that suffer from diagnostic error, as it has become top on the list for communities, because of concern for patient safety (Mascherek, & Schwappach, 2016). Consequently, mental illness was another area where practitioners and patients requires strategic planning from their statistical data to ensure that adequate diagnoses are confirmed, since patients are misdiagnosed when it pertains to mental illness (Mascherek, & Schwappach, 2016). The research questions primarily focus on the problem of medical errors and these problems can occur within any component of a medical setting or institution. Additionally, the research questions addressed problematic areas that pertains to what, how, with what, with whom, and where. These questions assist with identifying what occurred, how often, with whom regarding who was involved, and where regarding the facility. The questions, also, assist with referencing population(s) who experience the same or similar occurrences within specific demographical locations and when necessary include who were spokes persons for the patient, such as, caregivers, family members, or a friend. These important questions provided answers, since other individuals were involved in the decision-making process outside of the professional perimeter and those who are members of various religious affiliations. The latter poses challenges for patients and health-care professionals, because of religious ethical views of various nations and culture (Brügger, & Kretzchmar, 2015). The topics that pertain to international management theory provided information that focus on two main approaches that are faith-exclusive and faith-inclusive. Unfortunately, there was hostility within the faith-exclusive approach in some instances, because of resistance to integrating managerial practice views as only subsets of a nations' culture (Brügger, & Kretzchmar, 2015). Therefore, the construct focuses on medical errors and the role of team members in the decision-making processes to ensure that final decisions reflect best practices. This process eliminates bias that lead to conflicting practices (Berg et al. 2016). In addition, utilizing the qualitative method for research provides an understanding that was appropriate for achieving qualitative data to provide solutions for improving the decision-making processes within facilities or institutions (Berg et al. 2016). Incorporating the phenomenological method provided a description of the phenomenon that relates to everyday experiences for providing essential information that was important for formulating an overall structure for the research material. This approach was to provide additional information about the nature of the incident through the process of mediation to develop a grounded theory. The questions will identify the following:

1. Who was present at the onset of the decision-making process?

2. Where did the occurrences occur, operating room, emergency room, and/or adverse event facility?

3. When, where, and was return office visits recommended?

Subtopics

This study provides constructs with qualitative data in a cross-cultural context to synthesize evidence that causes complex interventions to address questionable areas about medical errors, by highlighting issues in need of improvement. In addition, this study provided further evidence that the quality of health care was continuously improving in comparison to data from the years of 2012 through 2017. The constructs for this framework summarized processes to provide essential information about various types of illnesses and treatments, to provide effective patient self-management (Feeny, & Santana, 2014). Additionally, this conceptual framework validated the level of quality care by providing criterion for communicating results between clinicians, patients and/or family members, which had an impact on the decision-making process and patients' engagement (Feeny, & Santana, 2014). This process provided information for improving results for managing clinician satisfaction, patients' adherence, and patient satisfaction (Feeny, & Santana, 2014).

The purpose for constructing a qualitative research design was to investigate the quality of care in the health-care industry, since there were increases in diagnostic and prognosis error rates. In addition, to concerns about behavior(s) in the health-care profession, because an article in the AARP Bulletin, indicated the health-care systems may be harming their patients by providing wrong diagnosis, sloppy practices, poor communication, lax hygiene, dismal discharge planning, knowledge gaps, drug blunders, dangerous doctors, outpatient black hole, buried information, clinician burnout, and small talk (US Institute of Medicine, 2015). The preceding information was about conditions and categories that contribute to causes for medical and diagnostic errors. Since concerns erupted in late 1999 when the Institute of Medicine published information that directed concerns toward the medical establishment, because there was an estimation of nearly 100,000 hospitalized patients who died annually from preventable errors (US Institute of Medicine, 2015). Therefore, emphasizing medical errors are the third-leading cause of death in the United States, after cancer and heart disease. Additionally, diagnostic errors received great attention over the past decade, but the concerns consisted of quantifiable problems associated with health care that pertained to infections, medication errors, and post-surgical complications. Although, these are important issues the argument here was the rising level of error rates associated with diagnostic and prognostic medical errors. Thus, concerns continues to grow over quality issues within health-care agencies and recommendations were made to take a closer look at factors that was associated with human error ((AHRQ) Agency for Healthcare Research and Quality, 2016).

New information indicates medical errors are now the sixth leading cause of death in the United States (US) and may be as high as 400,000, as the results indicated from a stratified random sample taken from 10 hospitals from January 2002 through 2007, in the state of North Carolina (Harris, & Peeples, 2015). Although, there was suggestions to improve patient safety no significant decrease in medical harm occurred. Therefore, continuous research can validate levels of occurrences and incidents that are associated with diagnostic and/or medical errors to provide a level of strategic approaches to remove barriers for solutions (Harris, & Peeples, 2015). Currently, researchers acknowledge that medical errors should rank as a third leading cause of death, per a study at John Hopkins Medicine (Allen, & Pierce, 2016). In addition, the research indicated the tracking system of vital statistics indicated important information was outside of the public's eye (Allen, & Pierce, 2016). Based on an analysis of prior research, the Johns Hopkins study estimates that more than 250,000 Americans die each year from medical errors. On the Center for Disease and Control's (CDC's) official list medical errors rank behind heart disease and cancer with each taking about 600,000 lives in 2014 and those errors were in front of respiratory disease, which caused about 150,000 deaths (Allen, & Pierce, 2016). To realize the impact of medical errors there was an estimation for the U. S. that indicates currently diagnostic errors occur in 15% of patients who received services from clinics and 12 million adults are affected annually, which led to damages, death or permanent disabilities (Khullar, & Jena, 2016; Khullar et al. 2015). Once again, medical errors are a feasible topic to research primarily within the geographical locations in the U. S., because approximately 80% of serious medical errors occur from lack of communication between health-care staff (Howey et al. 2015).

Learning models for change

Practice change was a sensitive topic, since it disturbs status quo, which has an impact on equilibrium, because of contributing factors, such as, evidence and context

(Aron, Boland, & Gupta, 2017). However, it can be accomplished through strategies that implement behavioral change, because it was important when it pertained to inter-professional education (IPE), which had the capacity to provide information for professionals from different disciplines to function in a collaborative environment to gain proficiency that ensure patient safety (Howey et al. 2015). There are health-care related studies on learning that adopted models for change from fields of management and business that focus on identifying barriers that pertain to challenges that physicians experience, during the unlearning process (Aron et al. 2017). In the meantime, studies have described various phenomenon and psychological issues that affect a physicians' ability to change and abandon outdated clinical practices to learn new information and procedures (Aron et al. 2017). The above information validated medical errors was a research worthy problem and with the correct theoretical conceptual framework it provides verbiages throughout the data collection process that was crucial for validating the findings.

Visionary conceptual framework

An additional approach utilized from a visionary was to verify the Quality Management Systems (QMS) of the TransCelerate BioPharma Inc., to identify potential benefits of developing a flexible QMS conceptual framework for proactive clinical research (Bergamo et al. 2016). The purpose for developing this approach was for stakeholders to recognize that the Concept Paper provides information that harmonized guidelines with International Council for Harmonization (ICH) guidelines (Bergamo et al. 2016). This resulted in providing clear expectations from management about expectations for QMS in clinical practices (Bergamo et al. 2016). This construct primarily consisted of areas that pertain to clinical development, issue management, risk management, TransCelerate, clinical quality, and knowledge management (Bergamo et al. 2016). In addition, radiological diagnoses are challenging, because most cases was influenced by clinical circumstances of patients, their history, prior images, biases, and many other factors (Brady, 2016). However, expert opinion can form the basis to decide if an error was made and can assist with confronting mistakes (Abujudeh, Bruno, & Walker, 2015; Brady, 2016).

Comparative research design

A first-time comparative study that pertained to nurse practitioners and physicians were constructed by utilizing a survey that pertain to evolving practices between nurse practitioners versus doctors' diagnostic reasoning in an acute tertiary hospital (Pirret, 2016). The comparative studies provided constructs to re-examine their bias against heuristics, regarding the frequency of diagnostic error through observational studies in outpatient care. The comparative approach focused on the dual-process theory, by highlighting the fact that it may be content and not the process that causes errors to occur, because of creating diagnostic errors through clinical reasoning, which maxim aphorism when medication was involved (Pirret, 2016). The results indicated both groups incorporated more intuitive processes when they paired with residents, both groups identified with certain maxims, and analytic processes triggered when required (Pirret, 2016). These processes are essential, because of the value and pitfalls associated with diagnostic errors can provide answers to who, what, when, and how while validating diagnostic errors does not occur primarily in a primary care facility. Previous studies verified nurses are as effective as doctor when it requires managing chronic conditions, injuries, and minor illnesses (LaGrow et al. 2015). The purpose of this study was to assess how to provide a comparison to contrast how nurse practitioners' reasoning abilities derive at diagnostic conclusions when it pertains to complex cases (LaGrow et al. 2015). Therefore, this approach

utilized a comparative research design that consisted of data that related to complex

think aloud scenario to assess diagnostic reasoning abilities. The participants were 30

nurse practitioners assigned to identify problems to propose actions to determine

diagnoses to compare between 16 doctors to present to an expert panel. The results

indicated there was 61.9% of doctors who identified the correct diagnoses, 57%

problems, and 34.4% were actions determined by expert panel (LaGrow et al. 2015).

These percentages were in comparison to 54.7% of nurse practitioners who identified

correct diagnoses, 53.3% problems, and 35.8% represented actions (LaGrow et al.

2015). However, the analysis indicated no difference between the two groups

(diagnoses 95% DI: -1.76 to -0.32, p—0.17, problem χ (2) — 0.00, p — 1.0, or actions

95% CI: - 1.23 to 1.58, p = 0.80 (LaGrow et al. 2015). Therefore, the results from the

comparative research design provided data that verified nurse practitioners' reasoning

abilities provided favorable results in comparison to doctors, regarding action plans

for quality health care.

Unidentified medical errors

Medical errors have been among the professions' concerns prior to 1999 when

issues erupted that directed attention toward the medical establishment, because an

estimation of 100,000 hospital patients died annually from errors associated with

preventable measures (AHRQ Agency for Healthcare Research and Quality, 2016).

Additionally, medical errors in most instances was not on death certificates (Daniel,

& Makary, 2016). Additionally, there were incidents where the cause of death was

not identified coded (ICD) to indicate human or system factors was causes for

limiting information on a death certificate (Daniel, & Makary, 2016). Furthermore,

information emphasizes that medical errors are the third leading cause of death in the

United States (US), after cancer and heart disease (Allen, & Pierce, 2016). The affordable Care Act was to establish a comprehensive health care reform system designed to provide patients with affordable health care, while expanding coverage, keeping cost at a reasonable price, and improving the health-care systems with the goal of minimizing error rates (Affordable Care Act Summary, 2014).

Type of diagnostic errors

Medical errors are composed of both diagnostic and prognostic medical errors (AHRQ Agency for Healthcare Research and Quality, 2016). Therefore, the primary purpose for this research paper was to encourage managers within the health-care profession to take a closer look at the quality of error rates to determine factors that are associated with human error and remove biases that are associated with availability or causes for harboring biases (AHRQ, 2016; Affordable Care Act Summary, 2014). Further, research acknowledged that more than 250,000 Americans die each year from medical errors, in addition the John Hopkins Hospital's medial error list validates that errors are the leading cause of death (Allen, & Pierce, 2016). The science of safety, now, communicates how breakdown in communication, diagnostic errors, inadequate skills, and poor judgment resulted in direct harm or death to a patient (Daniel, & Makary, 2016).

Although, there are no definitive answers from radiological diagnoses; however, the answers derive in most cases from or was influenced by clinical circumstances, such as, the patients' history, biases, prior images, and other contributing factors (Brady, 2016). In the meantime, the decisions can derive from expert opinion (Brady, 2016). Therefore, understanding and confronting mistakes has the capability to reduce errors (Abujudeh et al. 2015). Other areas where errors occur was during practice change when implementing new procedures, which occurs in clinical practices that entail learning new and unlearning old information (Aron et al. 2017). Furthermore, a grounded theory-based qualitative study provided information from a semi-structured interview with 15 primary care physicians at a Cleveland VA Medical Center. Results from the study validated practice change caused disturbance and tension when it involved providing evidence in conjunction with context, it cause resistance to change (Abujudeh et al. 2015; Aron et al. 2017).

Causes for medical errors

There are other areas where errors occur, which are in assistant living communities, nursing homes, adult day care services, and in residential settings (Bäckström et al. 2016; Harris-Kojetin et al. 2013). There are areas where clinicians fail to arrive at prompt and accurate decisions and these concerns have drawn attention from the *BMJ: British Medical Journal* (Jena, & Khullar, 2016). In addition, these are categories where conflicting practice occur (Bäckström et al. 2016; Goodwin et al. 2013; Jena et al. 2015). This provided evidence that majority of problems are gaps within educational processes from not focusing on clinical reasoning in areas where it was required, which heightens concerns for patient safety (McCarthy, 2015). Finally, content knowledge was the root of diagnostic performance (Eva et al. 2014). Additionally, information on the topic of heuristics to compare diagnostic errors as a comparison to validate health-care professionals' well-being was important and reveals causes for excessive error rates (Hall et al. 2016).

Other contributing factors that cause excessive error rates are associated with health-care professional's well-being and burnout when it pertains to patient safety (Hall et al. 2016). Moderate to high levels of burnout had an impact on the outcome on patient safety and caused unsafe work environments (Hall et al. 2016). Although, there was exclusions that were not limited to only opinions the material provided data extraction and quality assessments (Hall et al. 2016). However, under the category of studies measuring both burnout and well-being the majority (7/11) discovered both risk of burnout and poor well-being were associated with errors (Hall et al. 2016).

Summary

The information provided in this paper reiterates the importance of providing and maintaining quality care to prevent and correct errors, while providing adequate information to ensure there are no blind spots. The above articles identified causes for diagnostic errors that consist of failure to explain the patients' problem(s) with accuracy and having the ability to communicate and emphasize the urgency of the problem(s) to be addressed (Trimble, & Hamilton, 2016; US Institute of Medicine, 2015). During, this process it was essential to consider a research design that focused on quality that provided comparisons from a two time point cross-sectional approach, because cohorts such as, groups, class, or colleagues are unable to maintain, due to the death of a participant (Grossoeheme, & Kipstein, 2016). Therefore, the goal for these authors utilizing the longitude qualitative method for their research were to provide an understanding about chronic conditions, adherence to health-care policy changes, and the results indicated that longitude qualitative research can provide a powerful approach toward understanding complexities within the health-care systems (Grossoeheme, & Kipstein, 2016). In other words, by constructing data to focus on two time points for before and after policy changes or when there are situations when participants was expected to die are essential for qualitative research (Grossoeheme, & Kipstein, 2016). The authors' selection for this approach was to provide an understanding about individual experiences over time, to provide an understanding about longitudinal health care processes (Grossoeheme, & Kipstein, 2016). The goal was to provide data for constructing a comparative research design that provided data from the period of five years or less (Harris, & Peeples, 2015). The results from this qualitative approach provides information to consider from previous and current studies to validate complex intervention may be associated with qualitative issues or occurrences (Grossoeheme, & Kipstein, 2016; Higgins et al. 2013) and serve as a presentation to the IRB board for research approval. Thus, examining behaviors are essential for providing data that pertain to decision-making processes (McLaughlin, Eva, & Norman, 2014; Bihari et al. 2017). Furthermore, suggestions were in certain circumstances where diagnostic errors was misconstrued when it pertained to heuristics, because there were indications that content knowledge was the root of diagnostic performance. This research design presents qualitative data that was void of quantitative information to provide data to validate qualitative findings (Sarma, 2015). This research was designed to provide reasons that validated most human error in the medical profession presents evidence that there are relative prevalence and significance from this study that prove cognitive errors among doctors in health care are due to biases and cognitive errors (Allen, & Pierce, 2016; Bihari, et al. 2017; Harris, & Peebles, 2015). The results from the preceding study provided results derived from intern simulation sessions that focused on acute clinical problems. The results indicated cognitive errors identified by using a questionnaire based on the Likert Scales and technique that required think-aloud was due to cognitive abilities (Bihari et al. 2017). The teamwork and leadership abilities were determined by Ottawa Global Rating Scale; therefore, providing information that resulted in validating that medical errors are a researchable problem (Bihari et al. 2017). Recommendations were to promote "non-punitive culture" to encourage discussions for reporting errors that pertain to diagnostic findings to warn off legal and

disciplinary actions (McCarthy, 2015). This was important since the primary

concerns were patient safety and the importance of not overlooking errors, primarily

since diagnostic errors affect at least 1 in 20 U. S. adult patients in an outpatient

setting each year or 12 million adults each year (Garber, & Singh, 2015). The

information provided from researching this topic will benefit the body of knowledge

by improving the quality management systems (QMS) and develop a qualitative

framework that provides organizational information that identify measures, in order to

construct flexible data for clinical research (Bergamo et al. 2016). The results provide

clarity on expectations for QMS that focus on risk management and clinical quality

(Bergamo et al. 2016). Thus, making allowances to take a second look by reviewing

original protocols and assessing the impact it had on quality care by providing criteria

to correct errors, since content knowledge was the culprit of diagnostic errors (Howey

et al. 2015). This provided patterns for establishing goals to detect diagnostic errors,

which was crucial since there was evidence that 18% of misdiagnosed cases received

correction, although most went, undetected (Howey et al. 2015). In addition, the

primary goal was to provide information for gathering data, since it was to be stored

into categories for coding each category (Kulkami, 2016). This provide criteria for

checking data throughout the processes of editing information that highlight excessive

data, odd data, out-liners, and double entries to provide data that validated the results

(Kulkami, 2016). Medical reports was another area where errors occurred and

encourage fostering the thought *To Err is Human*, because it stems from the article

that addressed *To Err is Human*. Therefore, recommendations was made from the

committee who were involved with establishing guidelines to act toward focusing on

diagnostic errors, by encouraging health institutions to improve health-care professionals' education and training (Cohen, & Laposata, 2016). The authors acknowledge it was important to facilitate effective teamwork within health-care facilities; primarily, since there was tremendous dependency on electronic communication and many are not effective enough to communicate diagnostic data (Cohen, & Laposata, 2016). The article reiterated the importance of designating funding for researching diagnostic processes and errors; because it would contribute to the body of knowledge and eliminate minimum explanation about reports that are delivered behind the scene, while improving members' processes on the diagnostic teams (Cohen, & Laposata, 2016).

The concluding thought here was clinical practices entail learning new and unlearning old information. Therefore, the authors of this information elaborated on the challenges clinical practice struggles to unlearn. In addition, a study was constructed utilizing a grounded theory-based qualitative approach by interviewing 15 primary care physicians for 30 minutes at the Cleveland VA Medical Center the standardized interview was semi-structured (Aron et al. 2017). The results from the study indicated disturbance occurred with practice change; which was an indication that incorporating changes maybe a struggle (Aaron et al. 2017). Furthermore, a new equilibrium that incorporated practice change verified that a part of the struggle involved evidence itself; which caused tension between evidence and context the results suggested there was a constant influx of changes in clinical practices (Aron et al. 2017). An additional suggestion was for physician models to reflect change, since learning and unlearning is merely a punctuation mark (Aron et al. 2017). Therefore, unlearning models suggested reflecting as a multi-directional process that will remove resistance to change, which was a valuable contribution to the body of knowledge. Other areas that were noteworthy was information to determine the associations between health-care professional's well-being and burnout when it pertains to patient safety (Hall et al. 2016). The study found 16 out of 27 had a correlation between poor well-being and patient safety (Hall et al. 2016). All the scales that was provided in the study verified an association between one or more sub-scales associated with burnout and patient safety, furthermore the conclusion validated the high levels of burnout, and poor well-being was associated with patient safety. Therefore, acknowledging that nursing educators faces challenges when it pertains to handling complex medical care in real life situations according to a study to determine the ability to make clinical judgment (Bäckström et al. 2016; Brunaminti et al. 2017; Dominick et al. 2012; Garber & Singh, 2015). To validate their findings, the authors constructed high-fidelity simulation (HFS) to assess student nurses to determine their teams' abilities to judge by noticing, interpreting, and responding to complex situations (Bäckström et al. 2016). The results indicated low clinical judgment for students in their first meeting; although they were in the developing and beginning stages the study which validated further research was necessary to focus on health care experiences, age, and to assistant nurse degrees were rated second (Bäckström et al. 2016). Since, specific aspects of behavior have different characteristics, because of attributes of patients, treatment, and setting this was essential and the authors of this study presented information that validates the importance of not overlooking errors in the mental health category (Maschjerek, & Schwappach, 2016). Therefore, the study provided constructs to combine knowledge from prior research to provide existing initiatives and projects that defines priorities for patient safety, in the category of mental health care in Switzerland (Maschjerek, & Schwappach, 2016). The design for this study was a modified Delphi questionnaire, a semi structured questionnaire, and two around table questionnaires to gauge experts' opinion that pertain to priorities in patient safety in Switzerland's mental health care between May 2015 and October 2015 (Maschjerek, & Schwappach, 2016). The results provided nine pathways that consisted of medication error, diagnostic errors, non-drug errors, treatment errors, errors related to aggressive management against self and others, communication errors, errors that pertain to suicidal tendencies in patients, structural errors, and errors at interfaces of care where patients and organizations met and/or interacted (Maschjerek, & Schwappach, 2016). The conclusion of the study provided evidence that patient safety was important in the category of quality of mental health, per experts. However, it has been a seriously neglected category. Therefore, recommendations were that activities in research and practice were essential, because structural and diagnostic errors were on top of the priority list (Maschjerek, & Schwappach, 2016). This is important, since additional research in this area will provide valuable contributions to the body of knowledge. Moreover, information provided in the research was the major problem that attributes to the processes within diagnostic errors was represented by major gaps within the education processes for all health-care professionals, due to the lack of focusing on clinical reasoning where diagnostic reasoning was required (McCarthy, 2015). Concerns heightened, because traditional medical liability reforms are not effective when it involves compensating negligence or adhering to safety measures (McCarthy, 2015). The author emphasized further funding was necessary to provide additional research on diagnostic errors to improve patient care and to contribute to the body of knowledge (McCarthy, 2015). In addition, it was essential to require slowing down to provide intensive reflective interventions. Although, this process may appear repetitive it was mandatory, whereas, it involves reviewing the original protocols in a case (Howey et al. 2015). The authors' method focused on assessing the impact diagnoses present in an ecological fashion to validate the finding. Another design allowed participants to choose to review a case or not and another design was constructed to experimentally provide the case description that applied to the effects of absence or presence. The results presented the overall effects of the study that verified a small segment that consisted of a 2% increase for accurate diagnoses and few were revised (Howey et al. 2015). However, there were those who recognized diagnostic errors and corrected them, because the results suggested physicians utilize their abilities to self-assess and identify possible errors. Meanwhile, the realization was their ability to detect errors are not perfect, because there were 18% of incorrect diagnoses that was correctly revised and most of the errors went undetected (Howey et al. 2015). The study concluded as, it validated knowledge deficit as the culprit for the rate of diagnostic errors (Howey et al. 2015). Therefore, additional research can provide information to improve medical error rates; in addition to providing valuable information to assist with determining clinical changes that coincide with a literature review that emphasized the importance of communication and noticing clinical changes (Renz, & Carrington, 2016). Although, there are known negative effects of communication failure little research has focused on describing the etiology of communication problems that require interventions to improve quality care by means of communication in long-term care categories.

Chapter 3: Research Methods and Design(s)

The purpose for constructing this qualitative research design was to investigate the quality of care in the health-care profession, since there are increases in diagnostic and prognosis error rates that direct attention toward concerns about behaviors that are essential for quality care in the health-care profession. In alignment with the preceding statement was information from an article in the AARP 2016 Bulletin, which indicated the health-care systems might be harming their patients. The article verified the systems were providing wrong diagnosis, sloppy practices, poor communication, lax hygiene, dismal discharge planning, knowledge gaps, drug blunders, dangerous doctors, outpatient black hole, buried information, clinician burnout, and small talk (National Institute of Health (NIH), 2016; Novatzki Forte, Pereira Correia, & Pereira Da Silva Martins, 2017). Therefore, adding further credence that the above are contributing factors that cause medical and diagnostic errors.

The research method for this construct consist of methodological processes derived from data collected from previous studies of participants and interviews that derived from themes to provide a voice for the participants and/or formats that was aligned with the phenomenon. The questions are designed to answer why, how, where, what, and when medical errors occurred. Additionally, the phenomenological method provides a description of the phenomenon that relates to each experience that determine errors associated with each occurrence to highlight the results and contributing factors that pertain to the phenomenon, such as everyday experiences that relates to pain, trauma, and other issues that are associated with well-being (Giorgi, 2013). This method provides percentages to highlight areas in need of improvement to formulate data in a structured pattern for providing guidelines during the research process. The results from utilizing this qualitative method provided assurance that the information about the nature of occurrences or incidents was data that validated the grounded theories that related to diagnostic medical errors within the health-care profession. The beginning of the process requires gathering information that elaborate on activities of specific groups; such as those who receive services from clinics, damages that led to death or permanent disabilities, as well as, interaction, and communication between group members as it relates to phenomenological research method (Giorgi, 2013; Jena, & Khullar, 2016).

Theoretical/Conceptual Framework

The construct was designed to address problematic issues that pertain to accuracy, since suggestions indicated there were certain circumstances when diagnostic errors are misconstrued and were referenced to heuristics, therefore, indicating that content knowledge was the root of diagnostic performance (Eva et al. 2014). In the meantime, since there are circumstances when diagnostic errors are misconstrued and content knowledge was the root of diagnostic performance there may be circumstances when subject matters are referenced as *To Err is Human* and cause problematic situations (Eva et al. 2014; Garber & Singh, 2015)

The following information provided the theoretical framework for this qualitative study by providing data associated with slow or speedy decision-making processes that are essential for reducing error rates within the health-care profession. In addition, this framework provides the criterion for addressing phenomenon by removing isolated out-liners that are unusual events, since the errors did not cause harm. This provides a framework to assist with taking a closer look at data to identify problematic causes that increase error rates (Howey et al. 2015). Furthermore, this framework provided criteria necessary for identifying technological issues to eliminate high risk factors that stem from technology, high-risk procedures, and barriers toward learning (Eva et al. 2014; Ginsburg et al. 2016).

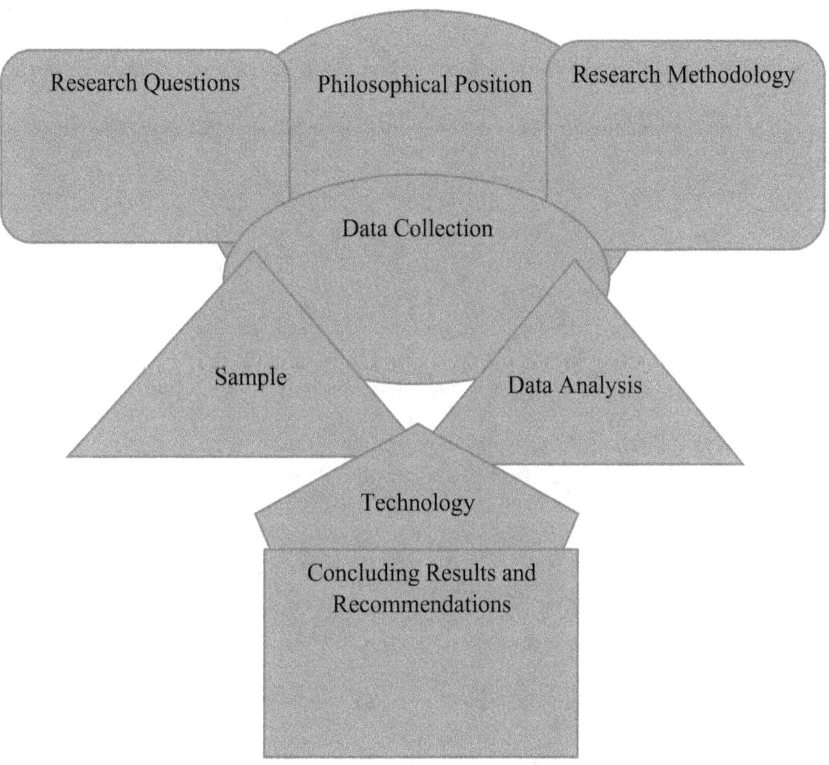

Finally, this process assisted with incorporating various aspects of hermeneutics to provide insight from online references to develop a starting point for where the data begins to the conclusion of the research on the topic of medical errors to provide reasons for various actions and/or phrases.

Population

The population sample was small to provide an in-depth comprehensive understanding of medical errors due to the nature of the study, since data came from online sources, only. This method provided an understanding about how individual experiences had an impact on the patients' outcome. When considering the population, the inclusion/exclusion criterion focus on collaborative efforts of health-care providers by concentrating on wellness visits rehabilitative care, chronic conditions, and new patients (Martin's Point Health Care, 2012). These are a few areas, which provide guidelines to improve collaborative efforts between health care providers and patients to ensure patient satisfaction (Martin's Point Health Care, 2012).

Size

The size consist of 10 or more research articles that consist of information pertaining to medical errors and quality care over a five-year time-frame beginning in with the year 2012 thru 2017 to determine if a decrease in medical errors had occurred.

Characteristics with appropriate support

The above strategies assisted with incorporating various aspects of hermeneutics to provide insight from online references to develop a starting point, in terms of where the data begins to the end of conducting research on this topic. The coding process links the research questions according to who, where, when, and what occurred with hierarchical levels for conceptual codes and additional levels for coding heath care processes, philosophical positions, data, sample, technology, concluding result, and recommendations. In addition, the research questions addressed the following:

1. Who were present during the decision-making process?

2. Where did the occurrences occur, was there referrals made, examples consist of primary care facility, operating room, and/or adverse event?

3. When, where, and were return office visits recommended?

The above are areas where examining behaviors was essential, because examining behavior(s) that address philosophical issues become necessary when gathering data that pertain to the decision-making processes, which require collaborative effort (Martin's Point Health Care, 2012). The above questions derive from the necessity to focus on the onset of symptoms, concerns, and about addressing the death of thousands of individuals in the United States within the health-care profession with the goal of improving diagnostic processes (Cohen, & Michael, 2016).

Recruitment

This process requires gathering qualitative data in a cross-language context, it requires synthesizing evidence that causes complex intervention for qualitative approaches to address the research problem. The goal was to highlight trends that are of consistent and inconsistent behavior(s) that has influence on decision-making process and lead up to events and/or occurrences to reduce excessive error rates. Therefore, constructing a flow chart to serve as a guideline assisted with gathering pertinent information for consistency and containment of information to accomplishing the following:

1. Maintaining structure

2. Provide consistent data

3. Gather multiple material from different sources

4. Avoid generalizing

5. The primary goal was to construct data to reduce medical error rates and provide a contribution to the body of knowledge

Data Collection, Processing, and Analysis

Collaboration during the research process occurred during the observation process by utilizing the material retrieved from online scholarly, *Academic Journals*, empirical evidence, *Medical Journals*, peered review, news articles, and university libraries sources. The goal for this qualitative research was to provide autonomy for philological historical insight, to serve as a guideline and focus on the concept *To Err is Human* (Garber, & Singh, 2015; Novatzki Forte et al. 2017). The concept has crept into society and has a hold on ideas that spread throughout cultures and cause conflicts. Data from this research provides evident that conflicts can occur, because of the errors. Most importantly, it was beneficial to interpret the correct meaning from information that comes from research data that involves health-care facilities with the primary goal of providing justice for humans by developing theories that provide evidence for qualitative measures to distribute throughout the health-care systems. This process required providing critical distinction between information that transcend from empirical evidence (Giorgi, 2013; Kulkarni, 2016). The importance of the hermeneutic approach was to provide an understanding about the nature of errors, various conflicting views, and the capability for individuals to adhere to instructions. Therefore, searching for information for open-end question was a reasonable approach for exploratory data collection that is unrestricted, since statistical data was not necessary to validate data in qualitative research to formulate the findings and in this instance, restricted data will not be included in this study.

This process provides answers to who, what, when and how incidents occurred to receive accurate data and conclusions. The benefit of utilizing the qualitative approach draws attention toward the urgency of reducing diagnostic error occurrences. This was important since there are committees that create reports who emphasize the importance of testing selections to interpret results (Cohen, & Laposata, 2016; Kulkarni, 2016). The purpose for this approach removed areas that cause guessing, although most treating physicians do not want to acknowledge diagnostic mistakes (Cohen, & Laposata, 2016).

Study Procedures

This qualitative study, concentrates on constructs, such as, data collection from observation of prior research of scholarly, empirical, peer reviewed articles; medical journals, and education materials to provide pertinent information on diagnostic medical errors for delivery toward the purpose of this study (Kulkarni, 2016). The purpose for gathering material on medical errors was to determine whether the errors are systematic or because of breakdown in communication and not individualized errors. Also, if they are attributed to high-risk populations that consist of men and the elderly who may require more physical examinations to decrease medical errors and/or coordination of efforts to improve communication among residents who are treating the same patient (Harris, & Peeples, 2015; Arnold et al. 2013). Therefore, the goal was to provide data for constructing a comparative research design that provided data from the period of five years or less (Harris, & Peeples, 2015). The results from this qualitative approach provides information to consider from previous and current studies to validate complex intervention may be associated with qualitative issues or occurrences (Higgins et al. 2013) and serve as a presentation to the IRB board for research approval. In order to develop a standard meta-analysis that provides a comparison between previous and current research with the goal of identifying and providing measurements to share from each study to indicate the effected size to validate the findings. In the meantime, there was little evidence that there was reform in this area, because data from both sides of the Atlantic suggest that despite numerous interventions to improve the quality of health care over the last decade indicates that the quality of care was deteriorating despite health-care providers receiving quality care training (Higgins et al. 2013).

The beginning process requires remaining focused on the importance of the committee's goal, because it assists with completing the requirements outlined in the dissertation process. This process ensures the completion of the dissertation manuscript chapters are align with the committee member's guidelines. This process ensures the methodological aspects and disciplinary components are aligned with the disciplines that are determined by the Chair, and Subject Matter Expert (SME). Weekly submission was required to assist the Academic Reader to review the Proposal and Manuscript against the Institution's rubric guidelines, constructive, and regular feedback.

Dissertation committee structure

The dissertation committee consists of the Chair, whose expertise was in research process, methods, and approaches. The SME's requirement must have a solid understanding about the processes of research, which consist of methods and experience to support doctoral candidates through successful completion of the dissertation process to ensure they utilized adequate references, such as, scholarly journals/books and/or articles that are peer reviewed. The Academic Reader must possess a strong understanding of NCU's requirement for quality research by demonstrating doctoral level research and teaching that meets the requirement to the specified program degree plan. The Chair, SME, and the Academic Readers have regional accreditation from an institution with adequate research and doctoral level teaching to support their students. The primary purpose of the dissertation process was to investigate a problem from a different perspective.

Assumptions

Assumptions evolve during the research process when determining if a problem was researchable and qualitative research can be an asset from exploring the best method for constructing managerial research for credibility, rigor, and trustworthiness when the topic was chemical engineering (Gapp & Stewart, 2017). The preceding three characteristics provide guidelines to move qualitative research away from positivist terms with the goal of utilizing the concepts, especially when researching medical diagnostic errors (Gapp, & Stewart, 2017; Novatzki Forte et al. 2017). Furthermore, this qualitative research was stringent enough to provide alchemy for deeper understanding to realize the value of further research and remove blind spots (Busch, 2016; Gapp, & Stewart, 2017) in addition to providing an understanding from back ground literature that contributes to further research.

Limitations

At this phase of the research, there are no reasons to anticipate limitations that will prevent further research on this topic, since current research indicates additional information benefits management, the medical profession, and provides a contribution to the body of knowledge. In the meantime, it was important to remember that the Institutional Review Board (IRB) must approve research topics and confidentiality was essential.

Delimitations

Attention was toward quality of care in the mid-1900s; however, there were conflicting evidence that occurred, whereas, some physicians found Patient-Reported Outcome Measures (PROMs) useful and others felt it was a waste of time (Feeny, & Santana, 2014). However, the importance of PROMs was to provide important information to guide chronic conditions and provide timely information for health-care providers in the categories of symptoms, emotional, and functional statuses (Feeny, & Santana 2014). However, there were a latent skepticism about barriers from skeptics about the patients' self-report and the unfamiliarity with PROMs (Feeny, & Santana, 2014). On the other hand, because of accumulating experience in a variety of clinical settings substantiated barriers have reduced, although there was latent skepticism about the primary care setting, due to chronic health conditions (Feeny, & Santana, 2014). The theory in this research was the implementation of PROMs and the incorporation of strategies for patient-clinician, clinician-clinician, patient-relative, and clinician-relative to encourage discussions about issues that are in the categories that improves communication and share goals toward better health conditions and treatment preferences (Feeny, & Santana, 2014). Furthermore, when research pertains to management, which covers every component of business practices, it entails developing theoretical data to investigate various input and output throughout an organization, to determine the organizations' efficiency. The goal was to highlight trends of consistent and inconsistent behavior(s) that have influence on the decision-making process that lead up to events and/or occurrences, in order to reduce excessive error rates. This required constructing a flow chart to serve as a guideline to assist with gathering pertinent information for consistency and containment of information for accomplishing the following:

1. Maintaining structure

2. Provide consistent data

3. Gather multiple material from different sources

4. The primary goal was to construct data to reduce medical error rates and provide a contribution to the body of knowledge

5. Avoid generalization

Ethical Assurances

Serves as a guideline to ensure protection for all human subjects by ensuring the highest ethic and scientific standards are in adherence to ethical principles outlined in the Belmont report. Their guidelines are to ensure respect for persons. It consists of an advisory board that was an external peer review committee. To ensure stringent guidelines scientific counselors evaluate information as they review accomplishments in comparison to a last peer review. This approach assisted with evaluating long-term objectives, innovation, accomplishments, and the relevance as it pertains to guidelines with the National Institute of Environmental Health Science (NIEHS) recognized as the Institutional Review Board (IRB) (National Institute of Environmental Health Sciences (NIH), 2016; National Institute of Environmental Health Sciences, 2017).

Summary

This paper reiterates the importance of maintaining quality care by preventing, and correcting errors in the medical profession with adequate information to ensure removal of blind spots. There are articles that identify causes for diagnostic errors that consist of failure to explain the patients' problem(s) with accuracy and having the ability to communicate and emphasize the urgency of the problem(s) to be addressed

(Abbasi, 2016; Hamilton, & Trimble, 2016; US Institute of Medicine, 2015). Thus, examining behaviors was essential when providing data that pertained to decision-making processes (Eva et al. 2014). Therefore, suggestions were made for certain circumstances where diagnostic errors was misconstrued when it pertained to heuristics, because there were indications that content knowledge was the root of diagnostic performance. The research design presents qualitative data that was void of quantitative information to provide data that validated the findings (Sarma, 2015). In multi-factor ways, articles that provide relativist attitudes and intercultural information are research worthy when it pertains to conflict management, which can occur when constructing measure to reduce medical errors (Busch, 2016). Whatever, the measures are when constructing qualitative research, it was important to utilize a systematic approach providing examples from scholars, peer reviewed articles, and up-to-date information to validate the findings (Colorafi, & Evans, 2016; Sarma, 2015). Therefore, there are various approaches when implementing different research designs. This was because there were two research methods that provided distinctive differences between their approaches, when addressing phenomenological psychology (Giorgi, 2013). However, they possessed some commonality, because the goal for their research was to develop approaches for qualitative research with the goal of providing justice for human subjects (Giorgi, 2013). The difference was noted when Mouskakaś referred to transcendental phenomenological approach and Giorgi presented and empirical-psychological approach (Giorgi, 2013). In the meantime, when it pertained to reduction the information was not consistent with Husseri's work. Therefore, referring to transcendental egos and when making comparison Moustaskaś referred to it as empirical ego, which narrowed the results down to transcendental consciousness, since bias was not present and represents an individual's own individualized view point about desired results that are important when validating findings and in this case results on medical errors (Giorgi, 2013). Primarily, since as of 2015 medical errors were ranked as the six-leading cause of death in the United States (US) and may be as high as 400,000, according to results from 10 hospitals during January 2002 to 2007 in the state of North Carolina (Abbasi, 2016; Harris, & Pebbles, 2015). This research validates that examining behaviors are necessary when focusing on decision-making processes. In this material, there are instances where researchers used heuristics for opportunities to observe behavior(s) that were associated with speedy versus slow decision-making processes (Busch, 2016; Eva et al. 2014; Giorgi, 2013). However, there were circumstances when heuristics indication was that content knowledge was the root of diagnostic performance and was misconstrued, therefore providing a valuable contribution to the field of study in the managerial and medical professions. The concluding thought here was because alternate views are associated with double-checking and different viewpoints occur when deciding to double check. To improve alternate views, requires a dedicated environment, thoroughness, and training. The results of the preceding study reiterates the importance of questioning, since there are limitations to processes, therefore strengthening the ubiquitous of the practice, because it was rarely challenged (Chreim et al. 2016).

Chapter 4: Findings

Results

The purpose of this qualitative research approach was to provide autonomy that pertains to philological historical insight as a guideline to focus on the concept *To Err is Human* (Abbasi, 2016; Garber, & Singh, 2015). This research received the approval of the Institutional Review Board (IRB) prior to beginning this portion of the research. There was proven factors that have validated medical errors are preventable, since human behaviors stem from the interactions between caregivers and the health-care systems (Zikhani, 2016). An investigation reiterated that accuracy was important for describing techniques and familiarity, because when it pertains to imaging background knowledge for medical image registration does provide practitioners with the main issues that cause challenges. There are numerous situations where medical errors and conditions required carrying out accurate diagnosis to provide assurance of successful treatment and one was during medical imaging registration, because it entails aligning images to provide a comparison between the patient with normal condition and those with different questionable conditions (Alam et al. 2017). Additionally, there are several different types of imaging modalities; each extract different types of information and each have their own features for extracting different types of information, because the imaging modalities has designs for human organs (Alam et al. 2017). This was important for providing possible solutions for guidelines that are helpful for developing new techniques (Alam et al. 2017). The purpose for utilizing such a technique provided benefits for fast recovery, in addition to providing crucial information to assists clinician with qualitative diagnoses to resect a tumor from the information on the image (Alam et al. 2017). This information validates the importance of interpreting the correct meaning from information during the investigation processes when it involves health-care facilities with the goal of providing justice for humans developed from theories to provide evidence that there was reasons for improving qualitative measures within health-care systems. Additionally, there was evidence that health-care systems may be harming their patients by providing wrong diagnosis, sloppy practice, poor communication, lax hygiene, dismal discharge planning, knowledge gaps, drug blunders, dangerous doctors, outpatient black hole, buried information, clinician burnout, and small talk (Abbasi, 2016). All of which are contributing factors for medical diagnostic errors. Furthermore, a case study that involved a dermatologist who realized after completing skin biopsies on two of his patients that when beginning the third procedure did not discover the instrument or any of the trays were sterilized (Ginsburg et al. 2016). Although, the health-care professional knew the risk of infections from sterilized equipment was low; however since blood-borne pathogens could transmit infectious diseases, such as, hepatitis and HIV transmitted diseases the professional experienced a dilemma that caused bias in decision-making (Ginsburg et al. 2016). Therefore, creating cause for conflict in ethical decision-making, since procedures required patients' to be notified about the incident (Ginsburg et al. 2016).

Trustworthiness of Data

The information from this research provides critical distinctions between information that transcend from empirical data as evidence to validate the findings (Giorgi, 2013). The primary purpose for the study was to focus on misdiagnosed cases that consisted of qualitative information, since quality was a major concern then and now. There were cases where Lower Respiratory Tract Infection (LRTI) caused high morbidity and mortality in elderly patients if there was delay in treatment, because it can cause exacerbation of infections. Therefore, resulting in providing

requirements for identifying its cause, because there are several causes for the

infection and it was important for determining if the condition was associated with

pneumonia (Durmaz et al. 2017). For example, the mean age for this research topic

was 73.3 years and each patient that were intubated was hospitalized for more than

ten days with trauma, cardiac arrest, pulmonary disease, and other condition, which

was a challenge for determining if a patient had pneumonia (Durmaz et al. 2017).

Since, patients in an Intensive Care Unit (ICU) had conditions that consist or multi-

morbidities more than one parameter was required and additional studies can validate

the value of the test that determines the extent of the infection (Durmaz et al. 2017).

There was extensive research to examine the cause of diagnostic errors at individual

clinician levels to determine how individuals' process information was valuable,

because the clinicians frequently use heuristics primarily with patients who had

common symptoms (Diagnostic Errors/AHRQ Patient Safety Network, 2017).

However, incorrect application of heuristics attributes to cognitive biases, such as,

diagnoses based on experiences with past cases, premature closure despite subsequent

information, focusing on subtle cues that cause errors when diagnosing, and bias that

lead to developing blind obedience, which was a major contributor for diagnostic

medical errors (Diagnostic Errors/AHRQ Patient safety Network, 2017). The goal for

this research was to unravel causes for diagnostic medical errors, in order to provide

data to remove future occurrences toward patients who undergo surgery on wrong

body parts, incorrect procedures, or procedures intended for another person

(Diagnostic Errors/AHRQ Patient Safety Network, 2017). Researchers acknowledge

that medical errors should rank third as a leading cause for death, per a study at John

Hopkins Medicine (Allen, & Pierce, 2016). During the years between 2015 and 2016 there was an estimation for the United States (U. S.) that indicated diagnostic errors occurred in 15% of patients who received services from clinics and 12 million adults were affected annually, which led to damages, death, or permanent disabilities (Jena, & Khullar, 2016; Jena et al. 2015). Additionally, approximately 80% of serious medical errors occurred from miscommunication between health care staff (Howey et al. 2015). This was an area where reasoning abilities are crucial, since it plays a vital role in decision-making processes. Furthermore, there was evidence from 16 out of 27 studies where well-being has a significant correlation between poor well-being and inadequate patient safety (Hall et al. 2016).

These author's informed us that adequate information was essential for improving error rates in the area of medical imaging as noted above, because errors has posed some issues that pertain to image registration, which was the most important task for an effective medical image analysis, as well as, the most critical step for several clinical application (Alam et al. 2017). The benefit of medical imaging techniques has led to the advancement in computer-assisted surgery (CAS) and radiotherapy (Alam et al. 2017). Other areas for concern was that high morbidity and mortality that was caused by Lower Respiratory Tract Infection (LRTI) in elderly patients and delay in treatment can cause exacerbation of infections; which requires identifying its cause, because there are several causes for the infection and this was crucial if the condition was associated with pneumonia (Durmaz et al. 2017). This study provided the means age in this research topic as 73.3 years and each patient that was intubated were hospitalized for more than ten days with trauma, cardiac arrest, pulmonary disease, and other condition, which was a challenge for determining if a patient had pneumonia (Durmaz et al. 2017). Although, extensive research examined the cause of diagnostic errors at individual clinician levels to determine how individuals process information was valuable, because the clinicians frequently use heuristics primarily with patients who had common symptoms (Diagnostic Errors/AHRQ Patient Safety Network, 2017). However, incorrect application of heuristics attributes to cognitive bias and diagnoses based on experiences with past cases, premature closure despite subsequent information, focusing on subtle cues that cause errors when diagnosing, and bias that lead to developing blind obedience, which was a major contributor for diagnostic medical errors (Diagnostic Errors/AHRQ Patient safety Network, 2017). Nevertheless, the goal for this research was to unravel causes for diagnostic medical errors, in order to provide data to remove future occurrences toward patients who undergo surgery on wrong body parts, incorrect procedures, or procedures intended for another person (Diagnostic Errors/AHRQ Patient Safety Network, 2017).

Findings

Below is information that validated content knowledge was the root of diagnostic performance and provide clarity to assist with taking a closer look at data to identify problematic causes that increase error rates; because there was evidence that when diagnosing, it was often difficult to determine the actual problem during early stages (Agarwal, Kumar, Vaish, Vaishya, & Vijay, 2017). The primary reasons were lack of awareness or suspicion by the treating physician (Howey et al. 2015; Agarwal et al. 2017). Furthermore, this research material provides information that focuses on medical diagnosis and prognosis error rates to provide evidence that medical errors occur during the decision-making process, which caused great concern for the medical profession. This was proven during a study that focused on transient osteoporosis of the hip (TOH); concerns stemmed from often delayed diagnosis, which consisted of 12 patients (11 male and 1 female) between the ages of 35-50 years old (Agarwal et al. 2017). The patients' was treated non-conservative with vitamin supplements, non-weight bearing mobilization, non-inflammatory medication, and bisphosphonates, because the condition was associated with an onset of hip pain. However, when it pertained to radiological findings the symptoms was out of proportion. The results indicated that awareness about the condition was important for clinicians to provide early detection to eliminate unnecessary treatment for other conditions that mimic TOH (Agarwal et al. 2017). Technologies play a vital role in diagnostic findings, because medical imaging technologies have led to advancement in computer-assisted surgeries (CAS) and radiotherapy (Alam et al. 2017). However, research validates it was not good practice to rely on a single image that was neither in the same period nor with a single modality (Alam ct al. 2017).

Research

Question 1/Hypothesis

In order, to derive at the findings this research provided answers to enough questions to become stringent enough to provide alchemy for deeper understanding to provide a realization of the value for further research and the removal of blind spots (Busch, 2016; Gapp, & Stewart, 2017). The questions focus on the following in figure 1.

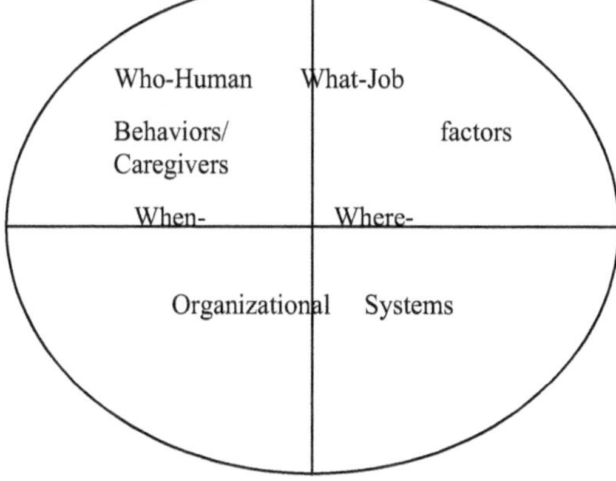

The above categories assist with highlighting areas for clarification about behaviors during the decision-making process to determine if occurrences occur in the primary care facility, operating room, or if it was an adverse event (AE), since these are categories that requires the most collaborative effort (Martin's Point Health Care, 2012; Zikhani, 2016). There were factors in this research that validated medical errors are preventable, since human behaviors stem from the interactions between caregivers and the health-care systems (Zikhani, 2016). Therefore, emphasizes was focused on human factors that were defined as organizational, environmental, job factors; and individual characteristics that influence certain types of behavior(s) that had influence on health and safety (Zikhani, 2016).

Evaluation of Findings: Categories

Who- There was evidence that 16 out of 27 studies well-being has a significant correlation between poor well-being and inadequate patient safety (Hallet al. 2016).

What - medical errors are the third leading cause of death (Abbasi, 2016). An estimation from studies published from 2000 to 2011 averaged medical errors that pertain to internal medicine at the national level based on 2013 hospital admissions. This approach estimated that medical errors was responsible for around 251-454 deaths that represented 0.71% hospital admissions in 2013 (Abbasi, 2016). Although, a health-care professional knew the risk of infections from unsterilized equipment was low, but blood-borne pathogens could transmit infectious diseases, such as, hepatitis and HIV transmitted diseases, which could cause bias in decision-making, as well as, conflict in ethical decision-making, since patients are to be notified about incidents

(Ginsburg et al. 2016). Guidelines are for disclosing medical errors to highlight mistakes (Arnold et al. 2013; Ginsburg et al. 2016).

When- This study provides information between the years of 2012-2017 from online research about the medical organizational systems, because as of 2016 medical errors ranked third for cause of death in US deaths. A study presented results that verified a small segment of patients that consisted of a 2% increase for accurate diagnoses with few revised, but those who recognized diagnostic errors corrected the errors (Howey et al. 2015). Knowledge deficit was the culprit for this study, because 18% of those misdiagnosed went undetected (Howey et al. 2015). As of 2015, statistics verified diagnostic errors remain an issue that is difficult to address; which has contributed to approximately 10% of patient deaths, along with 17% of hospital adverse events (AE) (McCarthy, 2015). Results from an empirical analysis indicated there was no solution to those problems that caused phenomenon between decision-making based on principles outlined for separation between faith and work (Brügger, & Kretzschmar, 2015).

Where- during 2016 information validated that in the United States (US) estimations indicated that diagnostic errors occurred in 15% of patients who received services from clinics and 12 million adults was affected annually that led to damages, death, or permanent disabilities (Jena, & Khullar, 2016). Diagnostic errors accounted for 17% of preventable errors in patients hospitalized and approximately 9% of patients experienced major undetected diagnostic errors while patients were alive, per Harvard Medical study; in addition, thousands hospitalized died every year, because of preventable medical errors (Patient Safety Network, 2017). A major error with long-term care was failure to communicate, which led to unnecessary hospitalizations for conditions that required long-term care situations (Carrington & Renz, 2016; Goodwin et al. 2013).

Additional research material validated that cognitive errors consisted of 90%, anchoring, and (75.7%), and premature closure (PC) was (78.6%) the study indicated there were areas in need of improvement (Bihari et al. 2017). This study indicated that medical errors are most when it pertains to preventable clinical decision-making, since most complaints were about emergency physicians whom delayed or missed diagnosed conditions (Bihari et al. 2017), as noted in figure 2.

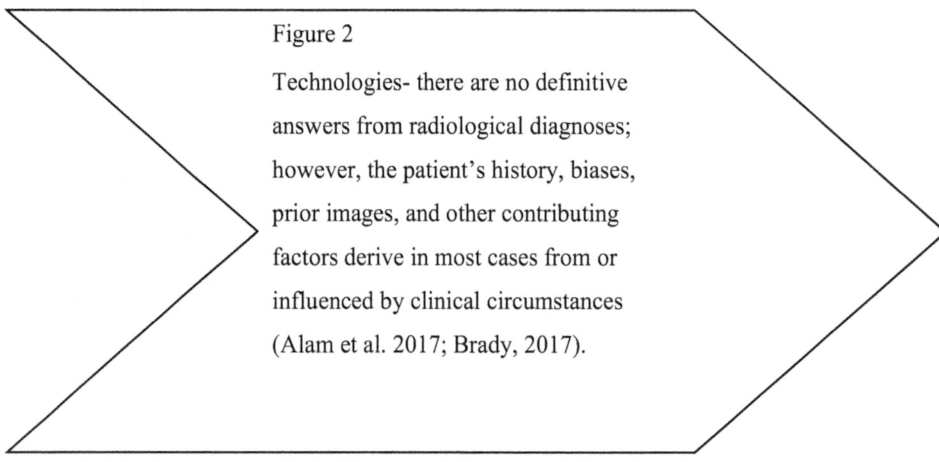

Figure 2

Technologies- there are no definitive answers from radiological diagnoses; however, the patient's history, biases, prior images, and other contributing factors derive in most cases from or influenced by clinical circumstances (Alam et al. 2017; Brady, 2017).

Summary

The above information provides additional key evaluation points that validates this research materials addresses the urgency to improve medical errors and that there are misdiagnosed occurrences. Furthermore, a study that focused on preventability of early vs late re-admissions where the measurements consisted of readmission with 7 days of discharge from the hospital and readmission that occurred between 8 and 30 days after discharge that fit into the category of late readmission (Davis, Dike, Doctoroff, Graham, Jupiter, Marcantonio, & Vanka, 2017). The median sum score was (8.5 vs 8.0, p=0.03); the re-admissions within 30 days received a score that was 15% preventable, 20% early re-admission, and 10% late readmission met the binary defined as preventable (Davis et al. 2017). There are similarities in this qualitative research that add credence to the concept that medical errors are preventable. Furthermore, it refutes the argument that medical errors are not preventable and cannot be reduced, because the major problem that attribute to processes with diagnostic medical errors are represented by major gaps within the education processes for all health care professionals, due to the lack of clinical reasoning when it pertains to diagnoses (McCarthy, 2015). This heightened concerns, since traditional medical liability reforms are not effective when it involve compensating negligence or adhering to safety measures (McCarthy, 2015). Additional information validates that biological aspects of behavior and social interaction can generate positive influences on health, because social determents and behaviors are responsible for almost half of premature deaths in the US (National Institute of Health (NIH), 2016). This research was not to argue the fact that with some health conditions loss of life is not preventable, but the preventable criteria must take into consideration the results of diagnostic findings, tests, and how accurate the test and results are identified in both diseased and non-diseased patients.

Chapter 5: Implications, Recommendations, and Conclusion

The research from this investigation validates patient safety was not on the medical profession's priority list for preventing medical errors. In the meantime, the reluctance to report mistakes or inaccuracies in the medical profession continues (Allen, & Pierce, 2016). Furthermore, concerns continued to rise over quality issues within health-care agencies, because they emphasize taking a closer look at factors that are associated with human error ((AHRQ) Agency for Health Care Research and Quality, 2017). Another study presented in this research provided a focused view on removing issues associated with diagnostic impressions and bias associated with heuristics, which had an impact on medical error rates. These impressions derive from placing undue reliance on expert opinion or total reliance on test results, however, the goal for this research was to focus on error rates by providing information that focused on patients, families, and the importance of integrity in the health-care profession (Patient Safety Network, 2017). Although, the study provides evidence that the quality of health care was continuously improving in comparison to data from the years of 2012 through 2017. The results from the study provided data that consists of qualitative information, since quality was a major concern for both practitioner and patients. Therefore, utilizing the qualitative approach provided additional information that was pertinent for identifying causes for medical errors, so the data indicates the quality of care before fatalities occurred from errors related to misdiagnosis and the level of phenomenon they caused.

Even though, an event study provides information to assist with constructing a theoretical probability analysis to indicate the level of incorrect diagnoses; investigations gathered from empirical evidence revealed what was certain or impossible to validate occurrences that relates to the quality of care that caused occurrences and reactions associated with the incidents. Thus, this study provides evidence that determined whether there were reasons to concentrate on eliminating issues associated with types of bias that would halt continuous research in this field, since a Harvard Medical Practice study validated that diagnostic errors accounted for 17% of preventable errors in hospital patients (Patient Safety Network, 2017). Additionally, this research focused on presenting data that provided pertinent information about events, situations, and behaviors with the goal of providing results to understand what caused the occurrences, in order to uncover, interpret, and reflect on solutions while investigating various aspects of those behavior(s). While focusing on quality improvement versus patient safety initiatives research indicated, there was a lack of strategic planning, per the most current report from the US Institute of Medicine (McCarthy, 2015; US Institute of Medicine, 2015). Due to the percentages of errors, the purpose for this study was to focus on and reiterate the importance of noticing clinical changes to ensure thorough communication was provided, because of the implication associated with medical errors and the statement *To Err is Human* (Garber, & Singh, 2015; Carrington & Renz, 2016). Even though, the above criteria received investigation concerns continue, although there are processes to ensure health-care organizations have procedures in place to identify diagnostic mistakes. As a result, this becomes challenging, since it was beneficial to interpret the correct meaning from information that comes from research data that involves health-care facilities with the primary goal of providing justice for humans by developing theories that provides evidence that improving quality in health-care was possible. Additional, goals were to provide a critical distinction between information that transcend from empirical evidence that validates continuous information provide criteria to examine the cause for individual clinician level diagnostic errors. AHRQ Agency for investigation focuses on who, when, what, and where that assisted with formulating data to answer open-ended exploratory questions to draw attention to the urgency of providing related experiences and descriptions that are comprehensive to ensure guessing is removed (Cohen, & Laposata 2016).

Data within this research verifies there are reasons for medical errors and answers questions about inefficiencies, lack of communication and/or bias as contributing factors for medical errors. Therefore, validating positive relationship among team members was essential, along with patient's capacity to adhere to medical recommendations that assisted with improving managing medical errors and procedures. There were circumstances when errors occurred that had an impact on business ethics, because there are many religious denominations whose beliefs have an impact on the quality of health care that relates to religious beliefs (Brügger, & Kretzschmar, 2015). Additionally, cultural theories are areas that require reiterating the importance of questioning intercultural mediation, because of limited research or questioning on conflict managerial practice. The article on this topic indicated that in a multi-factor way there are articles designed that consider how cultural relativist attitudes may stem from intercultural research (Busch, 2016). Therefore, validating that this research provides clarity for regulators on expectations in clinical frameworks to support organizations for evaluation purposes, tools, and resources (Bergamo et al. 2016)

Implications

Collaboration within this research occurred during the process of gathering material that was peered reviewed, news articles, and university libraries sources. It provides research focused on the implication *To Err is Human,* in order to investigate the quality of health care (Carrington, & Renz, 2016; Garber & Singh, 2015).

Additional implications were that the health-care systems might have been harming their patients by providing sloppy practices, wrong diagnosis, lax hygiene, poor communication, knowledge gaps, dismal discharge, drug blunders, dangerous doctors, outpatient black hole, buried information, small talk, and clinician burnout (Daniel & Makary, 2016). There was evidence from previous studies that complex intervention may be caused from qualitative and/or quantitative occurrences or issues (Higgins et al. 2013). Additional information focused on errors and discrepancies in radiology, because it was not possible to provide definitive answers from radiological diagnoses and in most cases influences were clinical circumstances, the patient's prior history, prior images, and other factors, such as, biases (Brady, 2016). There was errors that consisted of surgical complication that were not recognized, doses of medication that was mixed-up to the type of medication patients received, along with more than 250,000 American's who died because of medical errors was reported by John Hopkins Hospital (Allen & Pierce, 2016). Errors that involve medications, such as, antibiotics that was over-prescribed has drawn concern, because of acute respiratory tract infections (ARTI) that involved unnecessary antibiotic usage (Fahimi, Kanzaria, Kornblith, & Wang, 2017). Although, the association between diagnosis and antibiotic prescriptions were unclear from the standpoint of a study that focused on whether a patient diagnosed required antibiotics or not. The study provided valuable information since the study's population differed, because strategies included those patients selected who presented complaints associated with respiratory symptoms and fever instead of a final diagnosis; therefore, it required providing information to validate the findings from a real-perspective to better characterize patients with the potential for pneumonia by concentrating on the reason for a visited medical coding (Fahimi et al. 2017). In situations that pertain to diagnosing criteria for antibiotic may reflect a wide range of factors related to, but not limited to the patient, guardian, parent and/or physician's attitude (Fahimi et al. 2017). In addition, local practices and physicians' training can influence dispensing antibiotics (Fahimi et al. 2017). However, in one study patient preference was cause for dispensing inappropriate antibiotic and difficulty arose when there was no comment on the patients characteristics, such as, race or clinical outcome; because of cases diagnosed with pneumonia or ARTI requiring antibiotics, which could cause bias (Fahimi et al. 2017). Human imperfection can cause practitioner not to remain error free; however, the argument here was the causes for excessive or overlooked error rates that was preventable, because guidelines are established to disclose medical errors, therefore it require following guidelines to highlight diagnostic errors (Arnold et al. 2013; Ginsburg et al. 2016). Integrating Christian living and management toward national and international challenges can pose conflict of interest. Therefore, this was an important criteria, since within some Christian- theological approaches to business ethics there are certain management practitioners who practice separation between work and faith (Brügger, & Kretzschmar, 2015). When it pertain to cultural theories these are areas reiterating the importance of questioning intercultural mediation the author on this topic implied that mediation manageable cases designed from procedures that involve initiating designs for approaching conflict management was research worthy (Busch, 2016). Furthermore, medical errors occurred during decision-making processes and results verified that cognitive errors consisted of 90% anchoring (75.7%), and premature closure (PC) (78.6%), which validated there was areas in need of improvement (Bihari et al. 2017).

The research questions for this investigation was design to focus on patient safety throughout the medical profession, because there are many who received service in health-care facilities suffered from diagnostic mistakes (Mascherek, & Schwappach, 2016). Therefore, the research questions focused on medication, prognosis, mental illness, and diagnostic errors that occur within any component of a medical setting or institution, in addition to providing guidelines for addressing problematic areas that pertain to who, what, where, and when. The questions provided references from various populations for the importance of validating outcomes that pertain to consistent behaviors that attributed to medical errors. These are important questions since other individuals may be involved in the decision-making process outside of the professional perimeter and those who are members of various religious affiliations. However, religious ethical views can pose challenges, because of patients' nationality and culture (Brügger, & Kretzchmar, 2015).

Since, diagnostic errors received a great amount of attention over the past decade errors in the health-care systems has caused researchers to take a closer look at factors associated with human error (AHRQ Agency for Heathcare Research and Quality, 2016). However, an experts' opinion has the knowledge and capability to form the basis for deciding if an error occurred (Brady, 2016). In the meantime, this was an area where additional research can contribute to the body knowledge. Since, there were recommendations to provide reliable data for others to replicate so they can benefit from the results, in order to answer the questions that pertain to how and why an incident occurred (Ardhendu, 2014). The reasons for concern was prior to the year of 2012, research validated how and why medical errors occur by acknowledging in one case there was inaccuracies when diagnosing multi-drug pathogens and as greater networking occurred caused infections to spread rapidly (Jena, & Khullar, 2016). Further, recommendations were made to facilitate effective teamwork during the diagnostic process, educate, address performances, technological support must coincide with patient diagnoses, and suggestion were made to dedicate funding for research to ensure each error was identified and addressed (Cohen & Laposata, 2016; Cohen, & Michael, 2016). Additional recommendations are below in Figure 3.

Figure 3 Increase monitoring of how health-care facilities are diagnosing patients.	Increase collaboration between radiologist, pathologists, and health care professionals.	Encourage patients to share their concerns and get involved in their care.
Inform patients about their ability to access their electronic health care records and test results to ensure accuracy.	More training in medical schools and continuing education for making diagnoses can improve error rates.	Federal Agencies and employers urged to encourage others to learn how to avoid excessive error rates by reporting diagnostic error (Mercola, 2015).

Recommendations for Future Research

Progress in the area of addressing system causes for diagnostic errors has improved, because information technology has improved clinicians' abilities to follow up on diagnostic test to reduce incidents or delayed diagnoses (AHRQ Agency for Healthcare Research and Quality, 2017). However, a report released from the National Academy of Medicine in 2015 describing diagnostic errors as a blind spot when it involved safety. Further recommendations were to promote teamwork among interdisciplinary health care teams, improve patient engagement during the diagnostic process, implement error-reporting systems, and improve health information technology (AHRQ Agency for Healthcare Research and Quality, 2017). Therefore, providing information that is concrete, valuable, and remove the reliance on the statement *To Err is Human*, since such thoughts provided inadequate measures that overlook standards that cause harm (Gapp, & Stewart, 2017; Garber, & Singh, 2015; Carrington & Renz, 2016). Therefore, qualitative management developed the conceptual approach that can benefit qualitative management by drawing upon developments and advancements of other disciplines (Gapp, & Stewart, 2017). The approach will provide rigor for additional research and lead into triangulation for quality to understand self before attempting to understand the surrounding world (Gapp, & Stewart, 2017). Christian-theological approaches toward business enterprise reiterates the importance of ethical standards in business, whereas, Nils Ole Oerman, 2007, argued that in the business enterprise it was the main challenge of business (Brügger, & Kretzschmar, 2015). Additionally, empirical evidence exposed a paradox as it revealed Christian living, including some managers separate work from faith, because of reducing faith to application of principles that were ethical. Therefore, this process reduce criterion that involve ethics to a limiting-practice function (Brügger, & Kretzschmar, 2015). Thorough communication was essential and double-checking begins with the front-line practitioners and written, as well as, verbal communication was important to ensure continuous improvement in the health-care systems are free of weaknesses, since alternate views provide different viewpoints (Chreim et al. 2016).

Additional research highlighted the importance of changing institutional culture, since there was the necessity to warn off the notion that *To Err is Human* is acceptable from an article published in 2000 (Fibuch, & Robertson, 2017). Therefore, senior leaders and Board of Directors within the health-care system began focusing on safety as the core of quality of health care, because they cannot delegate the assignment to lower level managers (Fibuch, & Robertson, 2017). The article emphasized a just culture that provides a framework to follow and achieve an environment that promote patient safety that allow individuals to report errors without having the fear of retribution while focusing on the following in figure 4.

Figure 4 It requires creating a learning culture when applying new ways to establish practices are essential.	Creating a fair and open culture where individuals are not afraid to report errors.
Promote continuous improvement strategies by designing safe systems that provides requirement led by senior leaders.	Training individuals to manage their individual behavioral choices to improve quality care for patients. (Fibuch, & Robertson, 2017).

Before implementing the above strategies physicians were not required to provide oversight for balancing no blame in the workforce and they were not accountable to their organization, except to weak enforcement from their medical staff (Fibuch, & Robertson, 2017). Research on medical errors was essential, because it has the capability to provide criteria for improvement to encourage and enforce accuracy in areas that pertain to science, and practice of patient safety (Fibuch, & Robertson, 2017). This research reiterates the importance of an organization's structure, since the care teams are not always the cause for medical errors, nor is the individual providers and patients. However, safety issues in many cases begin because of decisions made by administrators, existing institutional culture, and environmental designs (Fibuch, & Robertson, 2017). The argument for this research on medical errors was to provide information that has capabilities to be referred to as Divine Intervention versus *To Error is Human* (Fibuch, & Robertson, 2017; Garber, & Singh, 2015).

Conclusions

Team members play a vital roles when it pertain to decision-making processes, because of their primary goal to focus on medical errors and ensure final decisions reflect best practices, in order to eliminate bias that lead to conflicting practices (Berg et al. 2016). Further, results from this qualitative research provided data from previous and current studies to validate complex interventions might be associated with qualitative issues or occurrences (Higgins et al. 2013). Research such as this benefits the medical profession and assist with improving managerial practices, as well as, contribute to the body of knowledge, in addition to acknowledging the importance of facilitating effective teamwork within health-care facilities. Primarily, since there was tremendous dependency on electronic communication and many are not effective enough to communicate diagnostic data (Cohen, & Laposata, 2016). Furthermore, the importance for constructing this framework was to formulate a grounded approach that emphasized the importance of identifying medical error to correct the errors. This systemic strategy assisted with locating flaws that identified causes that pertain to measurements and/or education (Jena, & Khullar, 2016). Therefore, verifying communication breakdown, poor judgment, diagnostic errors, and inadequate skills can result in direct harm or death of a patient, these result are caused from failure to execute, inadequate planning on a system level, or an individuals' action (Daniel, & Makary, 2016). Among the type of errors clinicians made were in categories developed in cognitive psychology that are classified with several types of errors, due to incorrect applications of heuristics and they were the following in Figure 5.

Figure 5 Cognitive Bias	Definition	Examples
Available heuristic	Diagnose current patients from past experiences	A patient with crushing chest pain incorrectly treated for a myocardial infraction, despite indications that an aortic dissection was present.
Anchoring heuristic that	This occurs when relying on	Repeated positive blood

consist of premature closure	initial diagnostic impression, despite subsequent information that is contrary to facts.	cultures with Corynebacterium dismissed as contaminants and the patients were diagnosed with Corynebacterium endocarditis.
Framing effects	Diagnostic decision-making unduly biased by subtle cues and collateral information	A heroin-addicted patient with abdominal pain received treatment for opiate withdrawal, but proved to have a bowel perforation.
Blind obedience	Placing undue reliance on test results or "expert" opinion	False-negative rapid-test for streptococcus pharyngitis resulted in a delayed diagnoses (AHRQ Agency for Healthcare Research and Quality, 2017).

Additional information validated clinicians are often unaware of diagnostic errors that involved them when they do not have the opportunity to see the results of their decision-making process (AHRQ Agency for Healthcare Research and Quality, 2017). Furthermore, recommendations were for teaching institutions to perform autopsies on 25% of inpatient's deaths, but few academic hospitals reached the benchmark (AHRQ Agency for Healthcare Research and Quality, 2017). Studies validated that many factors like human and organizational factors are most common on the list of medical malpractice and this was evident among all members of the medical team and especially midwives, because regardless of their skills they are capable of making mistakes even though error reduction strategies was in place (Beigi, & Khorasami, 2017). Behaviors are important to understand, because reflecting on the past provides an understanding about current experiences and predictions that pertain to future occurrences and it was essential for understand the relationships between information acquired during multiple episodes (Dominick et al. 2017). This investigation provides deeper understanding associated with improving behaviors, and mediate integration to enable inferences across experiences (Dominick et al. 2017).

The authors of this research provided pertinent information for strategies to improve quality care, because most people will experience a diagnostic error in their lifetime (Graber, Onakpoya, Schiff, Singh, & Thompson, 2016). Furthermore, within this category available literature synthesized to the present significant data for alleviating and addressing cognitive issues when it involves diagnostic errors (Graber et al. 2016). The final recommendations to consider was the World Health Organization (WHO) recommendation to bringing together primary care leaders and researchers from various disciplines to address common challenges, in order to provide opportunities to reduce errors (Graber et al. 2016). Inefficiencies, bias, and/or lack of communication was at the forefront of diagnostic errors and it was crucial to understand how to detect the system-based intervention plans at the beginning process that overlap the errors at the onset of diagnosis and prognosis (Graber, & Singh, 2015). This research provides important facts to consider, because the primary purpose of health care providers is to strive toward providing quality care and a just culture that was willing to contribute to the body of knowledge with the goal of reducing and/or eliminating error rates in the health-care profession (Arnold et al. 2013). An empirical analysis indicated there was no solution for separation between managerial practice and faith; no solution was for those problems that caused phenomenon between decision-making based on principles outlined for separation between faith and work (Brügger, & Kretzschmar, 2015). However, there was data that revealed practical problems associated with issues caused by separations, such as, conflicts, because of those who presented their own views as economic truth

(Brügger, & Kretzschmar, 2015). Other segments in health-care systems that require

improvement with quality care are nursing homes, because care within nursing home

facilities varies greatly (Goodwin et al. 2013). This information was from a study

conducted on a nursing home in Texas during 2006-2008 that focused on 12,249

newly admitted patients to long-term care identified by Medicare Claims as a

minimum data set of 100% (Goodwin et al. 2013). The information provided

measurements of care for over six months and the claims that were potentially

avoidable was over a period of 6-28 months (Goodwin et al. 2013). The conclusion

validated the efforts the providers devoted to nursing homes was associated with

avoidable risk in the emergency department (ED) and hospitalizations, because of

unavailable primary care providers within their facilities (Goodwin et al. 2013). The

mental health categories research provided nine causes for medical errors; which

consisted of medication errors, diagnostic error, non-drug errors, errors related to

aggressive management against self and others, treatment errors, suicidal tendencies,

communication errors, structural errors, and errors at interfaces of care where patients

and organizations met and/or interacted (Mascherek, & Schwppach, 2016). The

importance of this study was it validated that in the mental health category, quality

was essential and it was on top of researchers' priority list (Mascherek, & Schwppach,

2016). The researchers explored categories that have an impact on decision-making

processes, individuals who suffer from mental conditions, such as, ADHD and other

similar conditions from learning deficient; because rational reasoning can have an

impact on cognitive abilities, effect social rule, and memory (Brunaminti et al. 2017;

Preston, & Schlichting, 2015). Therefore, medical errors are a feasible topic to

investigate primarily within the geographical areas in the U. S., because approximately 80% of serious medical errors occur from miscommunication between health-care staff (Howey et al. 2015). The final results of the study validated that the primary causes of medical errors occur due to systemic breakdown in communication, and in some instance errors occurred, because of high-risk populations that consist of men and the elderly who require more physical examinations to decrease medical errors (Harris, & Pebbles, 2015; Arnold et al. 2013).

This current research provides information from examinations of cases that pertain to medical errors that received ruling from the Supreme Court (Cakmark, Demir, & Kidak, 2017). The information validated medical errors was one of the most important chronic problem in the health-care system, because treatment errors was the most common (Cakmark et al. 2017). Furthermore, the analysis validated human errors caused by induced human factors and they were costly. The article defined medical errors as failure to apply an intended operation the way as planned or applying the wrong set of actions that produce the wrong results (Cakmark et al. 2017). Medical errors are occurring even in developed counties and have become chronic in our country (US) (Cakmark et al. 2017). As mentioned above there are numerous reasons for medical errors and a recent report validated well-being has an impact on performance, because the data in the report validated that 20% to 75% of the residents around the world experience burnout (Bonato, Dewa, Loong, Rea, & Trojanowski, 2017). The national U. S. survey provided a report that indicated medical students and residents were significantly more likely to experience burnout with 44% of residents respondents reported high levels of emotional exhaustion (EE) 51% high levels of depersonalization (DP) (Bonato et al. 2017; Boone, Dyrbe, Satele, Shanafelt, Sloan, Tan, & West, 2017).

In order, to understand behavior and medical error a research was design to focus on nurses' behavior and factors that related to medical errors. Two reports published by the Institute of Medicine indicated every year in USA 98,000 individuals die because of medical errors and in Germany 100,000 medical errors occur every year, as a result of those errors 25,000 died (Dilemek, Korhan, Mercan, & Yilmaz, 2017). There was an 18% (270/327) increase in specific allegations against nurse practitioners in the past 4 years (Dilemek et al. 2017). Additionally, the American Association of Colleges of Nursing (AACN) validated there was a 28% increase of nurse practitioners who graduated during 2007 to 2010 (Dilemek et al. 2017). The research reiterated the importance of competency to have the capability to utilize the necessary information that was required to protect human life and health. Although, there was negative results different research validated the importance of nurses in terms of patient safety (Dilemek et al. 2017). Further results verified that nurses could prevent errors that originated from doctors and pharmacist, before patient suffer harm in a rate of 86% (Dilemek et al. 2017). A study for evaluation of patient safety culture in nursing services validated there was 62.3% of nurses who took training related to medical errors, 51% took the training in the scope of in-service education program in this study and it appeared that receiving education did not affect the attitude of nurses (Dilemek et al. 2017). However, another study-validated three-quarter of nurses received training that pertained to patient safety subjects and they found the information adequate (Dilemek et al. 2017; Arslan, & Karaca, 2014).

The importance of this research was to remain alert, ensure value, and produce as much accuracy as possible in the health-care systems. To validate the importance of an article titled Seeking value in health care: Have we reached the tipping point? In *The Journal of Health Care Compliance* that emphasized there are significant opportunities to improve quality of lives and the overall status of the U. S. and included contributing factors, such as, multi-determinants that involve one's social,

economic, physical environment, and individual characteristics (Cornett, 2017). This

researcher provided results about information that consisted of where individuals live,

play, and work; which are multiple factors that influence health care. Therefore, this

research construct was to help identify as many opportunities as possible to improve

health, well-being, and levels of medical errors (Cornett, 2017). In the meantime, the

argument here was everyone must be accountable and the attitudes of nurses revealed

nurses have expectations especially from managers and they must provide correct

evaluations on medical errors, because lack of management support about reporting

errors affect the reporting and provide negative incorrect information (Dilemek et al.

2017). Additionally, this research has highlighted many areas where

miscommunication can cause systematic problems and support the need for a standard

communication method that operate across disciplines, therefore, there was

recommendations to implement the SBAR Situation-Background-Assessment-

Recommendation) guide to communicate patient care recommendations (Hand, &

Stewart, 2017). The authors of this literature review validated that common barriers

was the organization's culture, hierarchical nature of the health-care system, the style

of different practices, lack of standardized process along with a complex care

system's complex information was what contributes to information gaps (Hand, &

Stewart, 2017).

Emergency departments (ED) pose the most crucial environment, since high

patient volume causes overcrowding, shortage of beds, staff, and shortage of space.

Although, this information was from research that took place in turkey the

information was applicable for medical services in the U. S. The solution on this

topic did not derive from increasing ED staff or beds, because the goal for their solution was to improve available resources by using value stream mapping (VSM), in order to become efficient and effective by providing a clear detailed map of the hospital (Bal, Ceylan, & Taçoğ, 2017). This study validated that the lean technique in the EDs combined with simulation models could be a very effective tool to reduce the patient value added and lead times in the EDs (Bal et al. 2017). In addition, the (VSM) value stream mapping method provided identification of the bottleneck(s) to regulate patient flow that cause ED overcrowding (Bal et al. 2017).

The above information from this research provided the capability for various components of the health industry to focus on continuous improvement strategies. This information has grounds in theories and acknowledges the urgency to monitor and improve the level of diagnostic error rates (AHRQ Agency for Healthcare Research and Quality, 2017). Every researched topic in this research has provided systematic and chronological information that reveal the percentages of medical error rates and what can have an impact on the percentage levels. The collaborative material are from online scholarly, empirical evidence, Academic *Journals Medical Journals*, peered reviewed articles, and university libraries sources. The goal for this research was to ensure justice for all humans that require critical distinctions between information that influence diagnostic errors (Giorgi, 2013; Kulkarni, 2016). Additional, reasons for this qualitative approach was to emphasize the importance of incorporating the hermeneutic approach to provide understanding for various natures of errors and conflicting views that has an impact on an individuals' ability to adhere to instructions. The benefit of constructing this qualitative approach has validated concerns and has proven that diagnostic medical errors was a feasible topic to research, however, most treating physicians do not want to acknowledge diagnostic errors (Cohen, & Laposata, 2016). The research material consist of information from the U. S. and other countries to validate that medical errors has real-world implications, although further research was necessary to determine whether medical errors follow a Gaussian or Power Rule distribution (Higgins et al. 2013). Furthermore, when medical errors occur to the level indicated in this research critical concerns have an impact on everyone involved, create phenomenon, clinical stress, and produce excessive financial burden (Jena et al. 2015). In addition, it validates errors occur because 90,000 deaths that involved hospital acquired infections were preventable (Abbasi, 2016).

Moreover, the information in this research identified problems that had an impact on medical diagnostic errors and answered the questions that pertain to who, when, what, and where to identify inefficiencies, bias, and lack of communication. Integrating Christian principles into managerial practices can cause problems toward national and international challenges, because of ethical decision-making (Brügger, & Kretschmar, 2015). Empirical evidence exposed a paradox that within Christian living some managers separate work from faith, because of limiting practice function since separation between managerial practice and faith was questionable (Brügger, & Kretschmar, 2015). Nursing homes were another component of the medical profession where research was done on patients who was admitted to long-term care focused on 12,249 patients who were admitted into nursing homes in Texas during 2006-2008, because Medicare Claims identified them in a minimum data set of 100% (Goodwin et al. 2013). This process provided measures of care over six months and the claims that were potentially avoidable assessed over a period of 6-28 months. The conclusion validated the efforts the providers devoted to nursing homes were associated with avoidable risk to the emergency department (ED) and hospitalizations, because of unavailability of primary care providers within their facilities (Goodwin et al. 2013).

The information in this study provided qualitative measures as a prerequisite for gaining approval from the IRB to further this research. The beginning process required remaining focus on the importance of the committee's goal and requirements for completing this assignment. This process ensured the completion of this dissertation manuscript and ensured each chapter was within the committees' guidelines. This qualitative research was stringent enough to provide alchemy for deeper understanding to realize the value of continuous research on this topic was necessary to ensure all blind spots are addressed (Bush, 2016; Gapp & Steward, 2017). As far as, limitations to prevent this study there was none; although accumulating experience in a variety of clinical settings research have substantiated barriers that was reduced, because of latent skepticism about primary care settings that involve chronic health conditions and little concerns about medical errors in general from prior research (Feeny, & Santana, 2014). This research validated that there was concerns about consistent and inconsistent behaviors and the necessity to evaluate various inputs and outputs throughout an organization to determine its efficiency (Feeny, & Santana, 2014). The importance of this study was to focus on improving communication and behaviors, because alternate views cause weaknesses and when double checking alternate views can occur and the results of this study reiterates the importance of questioning (Chreim et al. 2016).

9 787352 940314